Palliative care consultations in gynaeoncology

Palliative care consultations in gynaeoncology

Edited by

Sara Booth

Macmillan Consultant in Palliative Medicine, Addenbrooke's
Palliative Care Service, Cambridge, UK

Eduardo Bruera

Professor of Palliative Medicine, University of Texas,
M.D. Anderson Cancer Center, USA

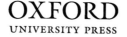

OXFORD
UNIVERSITY PRESS

This book has been printed digitally and produced in a standard specification
in order to ensure its continuing availability

OXFORD
UNIVERSITY PRESS

Great Clarendon Street, Oxford OX2 6DP

Oxford University Press is a department of the University of Oxford.
It furthers the University's objective of excellence in research, scholarship,
and education by publishing worldwide in

Oxford New York

Auckland Cape Town Dar es Salaam Hong Kong Karachi
Kuala Lumpur Madrid Melbourne Mexico City Nairobi
New Delhi Shanghai Taipei Toronto
With offices in
Argentina Austria Brazil Chile Czech Republic France Greece
Guatemala Hungary Italy Japan South Korea Poland Portugal
Singapore Switzerland Thailand Turkey Ukraine Vietnam

Oxford is a registered trade mark of Oxford University Press
in the UK and in certain other countries

Published in the United States
by Oxford University Press Inc., New York

Palliative Care Consultations Series Foreword

Professor M A Richards
National Cancer Director, England

Despite the significant advances in diagnosis and treatment that have been made in recent decades, cancer remains a major cause of death in all developed countries. It is therefore essential that all health professionals who provide direct care for cancer patients should be aware of what can be done to alleviate suffering.

Major progress has been made over the past thirty years or so in the relief of physical symptoms and in approaches to the delivery of psychological, social, and spiritual care for cancer patients and their families and carers. However, the problems of providing holistic care should not be underestimated. This is particularly the case in busy acute general hospitals and cancer centres. The physical environment may not be conducive to the care of a dying patient. Staff may have difficulty recognizing the point at which radical interventions are no longer in a patient's best interests, when the emphasis should change to care with palliative intent.

Progress in the treatment of cancer has also led to many patients who, although incurable, live for years with their illness. They may have repeated courses of treatment and some will have a significant burden of symptoms which must be optimally controlled.

One of the most important developments in recent years has been the recognition of the benefits of a multidisciplinary or multiprofessional approach to cancer care. Physicians, surgeons, radiologists, haematologists, pathologists, oncologists, palliative care specialists, nurse specialists, and a wide range of other health professionals all have major contributions to make. These specialists need to work together in teams.

One of the prerequisites for effective teamwork is that individual members should recognize the contribution that others can make. The *Palliative Care Consultations* series should help to make this a reality. The editors are to be congratulated in bringing together distinguished cancer and palliative care specialists from all parts of the world. Individual volumes focus predominantly on the problems faced by patients with a particular type of cancer (e.g. breast or lung) or groups of cancers (e.g. haematological malignancies or gynaecological cancers). The chapters of each volume set out what can be achieved using anticancer treatments and through the delivery of palliative care.

I warmly welcome the series and I believe the individual volumes will prove valuable to a wide range of clinicians involved in the delivery of high quality care.

Contents

Contributors

Jean Abraham
Department of Oncology,
University of Cambridge, and
Addenbrookes Hospital,
Cambridge, UK.

Dawn L. Alison
Department of Oncology
and Palliative Medicine, St. James
University Hospital, Leeds, UK.

Karen Bowen
Center for Palliative Studies, San Diego
Hospice, San Diego, CA, USA.

Lisa Punt
Addenbrookes Hospital,
Cambridge, UK.

Bristi Basu
Department of Oncology,
University of Cambridge, and
Addenbrookes Hospital,
Cambridge, UK.

Robin Crawford
Department of Gynaecological
Oncology, Addenbrookes Hospital,
Cambridge, UK.

Helena Earl
Department of Oncology,
University of Cambridge, and
Addenbrookes Hospital,
Cambridge, UK.

John Ellershaw
Marie Curie Centre, Liverpool, and
Royal Liverpool University Hospitals,
Liverpool, UK.

Sri G. Gorty
University of New Mexico
Cancer Research and
Treatment Center,
Albuquerque, NM 87131, USA.

Ben Liem
University of New Mexico
Cancer Research and
Treatment Center,
Albuquerque, NM 87131, USA.

Evelyne Loyer
The University of Texas,
M. D. Anderson Cancer Center,
Department of Radiology, USA.

Harmeet Kaur
The University of Texas,
M. D. Anderson Cancer Center,
Department of Radiology, USA.

Cheryl Palmer
Department of Oncology,
University of Cambridge, and
Addenbrookes Hospital,
Cambridge, UK.

Luis Padilla-Paz
University of New Mexico
Cancer Research and Treatment
Center, Albuquerque,
NM 87131.

John J. Kavanagh
The University of Texas,
M. D. Anderson Cancer Center,
Department of Gynaecologic
Medical Oncology, USA.

Sebastiano Mercadante
Anaesthesia and Intensive Care Unit,
Pain Relief and Palliative Care Unit,
La Maddalena Cancer Center,
Palermo, Italy.

Doreen Oneschuk
Division of Palliative Medicine,
Department of Oncology, University
of Alberta, Tertiary Palliative Care
Unit, Edmonton, Alberta, Canada.

Sarah K. Richards
Urology Department,
Gloucestershire Royal Hospital,
Gloucester, UK.

Alastair W. S. Ritchie
Urology Department,
Gloucestershire Royal Hospital,
Gloucester, UK.

Harriet O. Smith
University of New Mexico Cancer
Research and Treatment Center,
Albuquerque, NM 87131, USA.

Teresa Tate
Barts and The London Macmillan
Palliative Care Team Cancer Services,
St Bartholomew's Hospital, London,
UK.

Jay R. Thomas
School of Medicine,
University of California at
San Diego and Center for Palliative
Studies, San Diego Hospice,
San Diego, CA, USA.

Claire Verschraegen
University of New Mexico
Cancer Research and Treatment
Center, Albuquerque, NM 87131,
USA.

Charles F. von Gunten
School of Medicine,
University of California at San Diego
and Center for Palliative Studies,
San Diego Hospice, San Diego, CA,
USA.

Chapter 1

The assessment and management of advanced cancer of the cervix

Claire Verschraegen, Harriet O. Smith, Luis Padilla-Paz, Sri G. Gorty, Ben Liem, Evelyne Loyer, and Harmeet Kaur

Introduction

Across the world, carcinoma of the uterine cervix is the second most common malignancy in women, and is a major cause of morbidity and mortality.[1] In the United States, the incidence of invasive cervical cancer has steadily decreased over the last several decades due to the early detection and treatment of pre-invasive disease. In 2002, there will be approximately 12 800 new cases of invasive disease, and 4600 women will die.[2] The SEER data from 1992 to 1996 shows that cervical cancer mortality rates in the United States declined by 2.1% per year. In spite of the wide availability of cervical cytologic screening in the United States, 20–30% of adult women do not receive Papanicolaou (PAP) smears after completion of childbearing. Half of cervical carcinomas in this country develop after suboptimal screening, and up to 25% after misinterpretation of the PAP smear. Up to 30% of cases develop despite good preventive surveillance, particularly for adenocarcinoma variants. Because cervical cancer is related to HPV infection acquired early in life through sexual contacts, patients with cervical cancer tend to be younger than patients with other gynecologic cancers.[3] HPV infection is prevalent worldwide, and patients in developing countries, where this disease is a social catastrophe, are more susceptible to develop an invasive cancer after infection.[1]

The prognosis for stage I and IIA disease is favourable with five-year survival rates of >90 and 85%, respectively. The primary treatment of early cervical cancer includes radical surgery or chemoradiation therapy, depending on the stage of the disease and the histological type. Sometimes both, are used depending on the response to the initial treatment.[4]

The most significant advance in the treatment of cervical cancer has been the introduction of chemotherapy given at the time of pelvic radiation therapy. Five prospective studies, involving 1912 women with cervical cancer, showed that platinum-based chemotherapy, when given concurrently with radiation therapy, prolongs survival in women with locally advanced cervical cancer, stages IB2, bulky IIA, and IIB–IVA. Concurrent cisplatin or platin-containing regimens reduce the risk of recurrence by 30 to 50%.[5] It takes considerable time to recover physically, sexually, and emotionally from these therapeutic procedures.[6]

For patients with advanced disease, the risk of metastases, and the risk of local recurrence remains substantial,[4] and the diagnosis of persistent or recurrent disease can be devastating. Specific clinical problems arise in the care of patients with advanced cervical cancers. It is virtually impossible to predict how long a patient will live after the diagnosis of recurrence but, on average, the lifespan ranges from six months to two years.[4] During this time, most patients become symptomatic and will require good palliative care to preserve quality of life.

Patterns of failure of primary treatment

Cervical cancer may relapse either locally or with distant metastases, approximately half the patients will present with a combination of local and disseminated disease.[4]

Local failure

The most common pattern of recurrence is local failure (Figs 1.1 and 1.2), which may happen after surgery or after radiotherapy. Local failure after surgery may often be salvaged by radiotherapy with or without concurrent

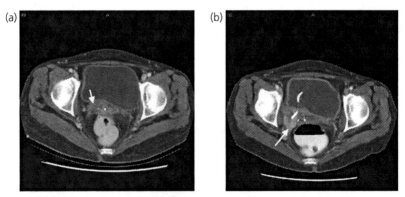

Fig. 1.1 A 54-year-old with poorly differentiated stage IV A squamous carcinoma of the cervix treated with chemo-radiation responded with decrease in size of mass. (a) Recurrence extending to right pelvic side-wall (*arrow*) was diagnosed seven months after completion of radiation. (b) Post-contrast axial CT images show enhancing recurrent tumour abutting right obturator internus muscle (*arrow*).

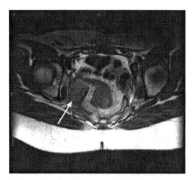

Fig. 1.2 A 32-year-old with cervical adenocarcinoma stage IB1 treated with radical hysterectomy followed by radiation. She developed a central recurrence, which was treated with anterior pelvic exenteration. Subsequently a right side-wall recurrence was found after 7 months. Axial T2 weighted images show hyperintense mass (*arrow*) inseparable from right obturator internus muscle.

chemotherapy. There are three types of local failure after treatment with a radiotherapy-based regimen.

Central recurrence

Central failure, which is failure within the radiated field, is relatively uncommon for early stage disease (7% stage IB and IIA, 15% stage IIB). Of patients with more advanced disease including stages III and IVA, 20–35% recur within the radiated field. Central recurrence is used to denote recurrence within the vagina, cervix, uterus, and/or parametrium, but without extension into the pelvic side-wall (Fig. 1.3). The only hope of cure for a woman with central recurrence is pelvic exenteration.[7] Depending upon the criteria used to screen patients for this procedure, the cure rate following pelvic exenteration is 25–80%. The likelihood of cure is dependent upon a number of factors, including the stage at diagnosis, local extent of disease, and the time between initial diagnosis and the documentation of recurrence. Persistent disease within six months of therapy has a poorer prognosis, as does recurrence in patients with a history of pelvic sidewall disease (stage III), or bladder and/or rectal involvement (stage IVA) (Fig. 1.4). Occasionally, patients may have pre-existing hydronephrosis, or the ureteral obstruction may be at the bladder trigone; in such cases, a work-up for exenteration may be reasonable. Patients with previous documentation of pelvic or para-aortic metastases are less likely to have central recurrence as the only source of disease. There is no data to support the benefit of palliative exenteration, which does not significantly improve the quality or length of life. A clinical workup should be done to rule out distant metastases, and includes chest, abdomen, and pelvic MRIs or CT scans, bone scan, examination under

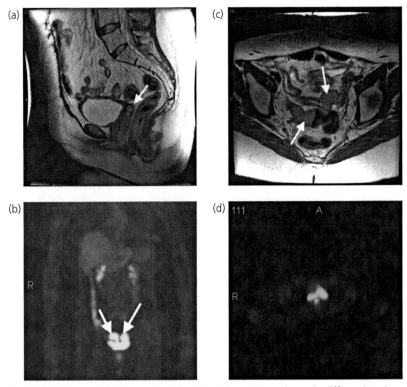

Fig. 1.3 A 49-year-old diagnosed with clinical stage IB1 and poorly differentiated squamous cell carcinoma. A radical hysterectomy was performed followed by chemoradiation. On follow-up a sagittal T2 weighted image showed a nodular hyperintense focus (*arrow*) at the vaginal apex (a) that corresponded to an area of increased uptake seen posterior to the bladder (*b*) on an axial PET image (*arrow*). (c) Axial T2 weighted images also showed two areas of eccenteric thickening of the sigmoid colon that were felt to represent peritoneal implants. (d) A coronal PET scan showed increased uptake in both these areas (*arrows*). The patient subsequently underwent a pelvic exenteration.

anaesthesia, and perhaps a scalene fat pad biopsy.[7] Evaluation of extent of tumour is best obtained with MR imaging. MRI is superior to CT in both the diagnosis and staging of locally recurrent disease. The excellent soft-tissue resolution and multiplaner capabilities of this technique enable definition of tumour and its relationship to the pelvic side-wall, diaphragm, bladder and rectum. CT and MRI are comparable in the evaluation of distant metastases, particularly adenopathy.

Excellent surgical training together with the availability of critical care units has significantly enhanced the probability of patients surviving pelvic

(a) 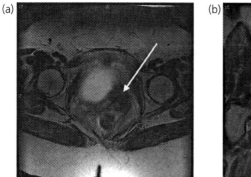 (b)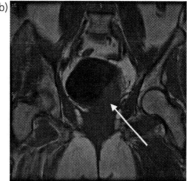

Fig. 1.4 A 32-year-old with stage IB1 squamous carcinoma of the cervix treated with radical hysterectomy. She presented with pain in the left posterior leg and leg swelling: (a) axial T2 weighted images show hyperintense mass invading bladder (*arrow*); (b) coronal T1 weighted images show tumour invading the bladder and levator ani (*arrow*).

exenteration. The extent of exenterative surgery depends upon the location of the tumour. For patients with small lesions confined to the anterior urogenital compartment, anterior pelvic exenteration may be sufficient. This procedure includes *en bloc* resection of uterus, parametrium (uterosacral and cardinal ligaments), and bladder, with the creation of a neobladder using a detached segment of ileum, transverse colon, sigmoid colon, or detubularized caecum and ascending colon. A reservoir that will hold 500–750 cc of urine can be constructed, and the patient learns to self-catheterize through a small stoma connected to the terminal ileum or to the appendix through the umbilicus or lower abdomen. Continent procedures are associated with longer operative times, higher peri-operative complication rates, and higher rates of surgical re-operation. However, they may reduce the incidence of chronic renal failure, which has been reported to occur in up to 10% of long-term survivors.[8]

Posterior pelvic exenteration involves the removal of the rectum *en bloc* with mullerian structures. Anterior and posterior pelvic exenteration may be supralevator, or infralevator. Supralevator exenteration, with preservation of part of the vagina, the clitoris, urethra, and anal sphincter, may be possible when disease does not extend into the bladder trigone, the lower vagina, or lower rectum. In these cases, posterior exenteration consists of a low anterior resection with primary re-anastomosis to non-radiated sigmoid colon. When disease extends into the lower third of the vagina, the paracolpos, bladder trigone, or rectum, the procedure may require removal of the urethra, clitoris, the entire vagina, and the anus/anal sphincter. In such cases, patients will require a permanent colostomy. Restoration of the pelvic floor may be accomplished by the use of myocutaneous flaps, most commonly involving use of the gracilis muscle. Transverse or vertical rectus abdominis myocutaneous flaps from the anterior abdomen have highly reliable blood supply, and better fit in the pelvis following preservation of the bladder or rectum.

Short-term complications of pelvic exenteration These include blood loss, typically requiring multiple transfusions, infection, ureteral anastomotic leaks (15–35%), peristomal complication, intestinal obstruction, fistula, necrosis of myocutaneous flaps, and death (3–10%).

Long-term complications of pelvic exenteration These include recurrent intestinal obstruction, diarrhea, malabsorption of fat-soluble vitamins resulting in coagulation disorders and megaloblastic anaemia, and weight loss. The psychological ramifications of pelvic exenteration have received little attention. Depression over real and perceived sexual attractiveness because of the presence of stomas, and with loss of the uterus and vagina, is common.

Alternatives to pelvic exenteration For patients whose disease is not resectable because of concurrent medical conditions, or for patients who refuse exenteration, re-irradiation could be offered. In this case, it is imperative to have a long discussion about the increase in complications and the low probability of cure. Tissues that have been previously irradiated do not have the same tolerance as those that have not. One must also review very carefully the details of the initial therapy, paying close attention to the energy of the X-rays, volume treated, total doses used (including external beam and implant), and the time that has elapsed since initial treatment. Once the decision to deliver radiation therapy is made, the volume to be treated and the dose must be considered. In general, limited volumes should be treated with a limited dose (40–45 Gy in 1.8 Gy fractions).[9] Care should be taken to limit the dose to normal structures as much as possible. A novel approach may be to use newer external beam radiation therapy techniques, such as intensity modulated radiotherapy, to deliver a higher dose to the recurrent tumour and a lower dose to normal tissues. Another possibility is to treat these patients with brachytherapy.[9] This approach would be better for tumours that are small and well-circumscribed.

Peripheral recurrence outside the radiation field

In some cases, the local failure occurs just at the periphery of the radiated field (Fig. 1.5). This problem can be cured in a fair number of patients, if it is properly diagnosed. MR imaging is the best non-invasive modality for diagnosis of recurrent disease. This technique has a high sensitivity but low specificity, as ooedema and fibrosis induced by radiation may mimic recurrence. The presence

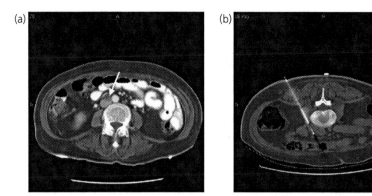

Fig. 1.5 A 54-year-old with stage IVA cervical cancer responded locally to radiation therapy, however relapsed in the retroperitoneum: (a) axial contrast-enhanced CT scan shows necrotic retroperitoneal adenopathy (*arrow*); (b) CT-guided biopsy confirmed metastatic disease.

of a baseline post-treatment scan improves the likelihood for early diagnosis and should be obtained in all patients. Newer techniques such as dynamic MR imaging and PET scanning have also improved accuracy and specificity (Fig. 1.3).

Review of the radiation fields is mandatory, to determine the correlation with the anatomical shape of the recurrent tumour, and to determine the safety of additional radiation. Because of the 1999 NIH announcement on using chemo-radiation for patients with poor prognostic factors, the addition of chemotherapy to this type of radiotherapy could be recommended. Current chemotherapy sensitization regimens include weekly cisplatin at 40 mg/m^2/week for six doses, or a combination of cisplatin 75 mg/m^2 on day 1 and 29, and a 96-h continuous infusion of 5 fluorouracil at 500 mg/m^2/day starting on day 1 and repeated on day 29.[5] Many other chemotherapy combinations for radiotherapy sensitization are currently being tested in controlled studies.

Peripheral recurrence inside the radiation field

Unless the patient is a candidate for pelvic exenteration, recurrence within the field of radiation is incurable. The triad of hydronephrosis, leg oedema, and pain almost always denotes unresectable pelvic side-wall recurrence. Hemipelvectomy has been attempted in these patients, but there is no evidence that this extremely morbid operative procedure enhances survival in these women, and it should not be performed.

There is no FDA-approved chemotherapy for advanced or recurrent cancer of the cervix. Response rates to single agent chemotherapy in phase II trials, other than that of cisplatin, have been 10–15%, and to combination chemotherapy, 35–60%.[10] In most series, responses are usually partial or transient, with no improvement in long term survivals.[10] Cisplatin is the single most effective chemotherapeutic agent in the treatment of recurrent cervical cancer, with reported response rates as high as 30%. However, response rates within radiated tissues are much poorer, 15% or less. For patients who do respond, the response duration is in the order of 4–6 months, and it is uncertain that chemotherapy increases the life-expectancy of these patients. Later in this chapter, the indications for chemotherapy in recurrence will be discussed in greater detail.

Presenting symptoms

The presenting symptoms of pelvic recurrent disease depend on the location of the tumour.

They may include progressive and severe pain from nerve compression. Obturator nerve involvement is manifested by anterior leg pain, and sciatic nerve involvement, by posterior thigh pain.

Approximately 14% of patients develop bone metastases that may result in pain, fractures, and, if involving the spine, cauda equina syndrome. Rarely, cord compression may develop, causing leg weakness, and severe pain.

Bilateral ureteral obstruction causes renal failure.

Leg oedema may result from lymphatic or venous obstruction.

Cervical carcinoma is associated with hypercoagulability and thrombocytosis, which increase the risk of deep venous thrombosis and pulmonary embolus.

Patients may experience a foul discharge from necrotic fungation of tumour at the top of the vagina.

Recurrent infections, including fungemia, are not uncommon.

Tumour may erode into the uterine and pelvic vessels resulting in a haemorrhage.

Symptom control for these problems is addressed in more detail in other chapters.

Goals of treatment in recurrent disease

The treatment of patients with recurrent cervical cancer should concentrate on palliative care. It is extremely important to communicate effectively with these patients in order to obtain an accurate description of the symptoms they are experiencing and to understand their priorities for the time that is left. It is essential to perform a good physical and radiological evaluation and to have extensive discussions with the patient to determine the best course of therapy; any treatment, including chemotherapy, in this situation is for palliation only.

Management of the complications of recurrent disease

Pain and fistulae The management of pain and fistulae, two major problems in advanced cervical malignancy, is discussed in Chapters 4 and 6. The vulva may specifically become excoriated and painful, and intensive local care is required to keep the area dry and the skin healthy. Perineal skin should be washed with soap or almond oil if the lesions are painful, and dried thoroughly. Perineal soaking can be useful. A protective cream containing zinc oxide should be applied. If the area looks infected, a swab should be taken for culture, and antibiotherapy directed against the infecting organisms initiated. If the fistula opens to the abdominal wall, bagging may be needed; an ostomy nurse should then be consulted. Octreotide also has a place in the treatment of diarrhoea caused by an enterocolic fistula.[11]

Renal failure Renal failure by compression of the ureters always poses an ethical dilemma. Haemodialysis is usually inappropriate. If a nephrostomy or a ureteral stent placement is feasible, re-establishing the urine flow may prolong the patient's life for an average of 4 months. If the quality of life is poor, because of intractable pain or other complications of the cancer, an end-of-life discussion should be held with the patient, because abstaining from opening the urinary conduits may be the better option. Prolonging the patient's life, may not be the best approach in a terminally ill patient. Patients most likely to benefit from urinary diversion are those for whom therapeutic options are available for the recurrent cervical malignancy. Therefore, stenting of the ureter or placement of a nephrostomy should never be a decision made without full reflection on the possible consequences. In a patient with good quality of life, urinary flow should be re-established, so that the patient could enjoy a few more months of life. Unilateral ureteral compression should probably be left untreated to avoid the complications from the placement of a stent or a nephrostomy (chronic infections, leaks, re-obstruction, or pain). Patients can live a normal life with one kidney.[12]

Vascular obstruction Venous thrombosis by compression of the iliac veins is one of the most frequent early signs of cancer progression. Typically, patients present with a swollen leg, resulting from a compression of the iliac vein by the growing cancer. Heparin anticoagulation improves local venous flow by preventing further clot adhesion and by decreasing the concomitant inflammation. Often, when the compression is mechanical, the leg remains swollen, causing additional patient discomfort and limitation of activity. Compression hoses are useful to relieve the heavy sensation of which some patients complain. Anticoagulation can be achieved by low molecular weight heparins, followed by long-term warfarin therapy. Most patients may require life-long anticoagulation, as the primary cause of the phlebitis is unlikely to resolve.

See Chapter 9 for a detailed discussion on management of thrombosis.

Lympho-oedema Lympho-oedema is a complication of combined treatment with surgery and radiotherapy of primary cervical cancer or caused by tumour emboli in the remaining lymphatic vessels. The International Society for Lymphology assessment criteria are based on skin condition, including the degree of fibrosis and the extent of pitting of the oedema (more fibrosis and less pitting indicates a worse condition).[13] Great care needs to be taken to avoid cuts or fungal infection of the feet, which could be a port of entry for skin pathogens. Patients with lympho-oedema have a tendency to develop infectious cellulitis. A physical therapist specialized in lympho-oedema therapy should be consulted for lymph drainage by the massage technique of effleurage and for mechanical compression with external graded compression bandaging, which may help reduce the symptoms of pain and body image distortion.

Tumour necrosis One common problem of pelvic recurrence is necrotic fungation of the tumour eroding the top of the vagina, causing bad odours (smell of rotting flesh), haemorrhage, and/or infections. Bad odours and infections are treated by vaginal hygiene, with very gentle douching containing diluted peroxide, vinegar, or just plain normal saline. A 2-week course of clindamycin, 300 mg orally three times a day may be attempted, as it often will control the necrotic odour. Topical metronidazole (0.75 or 0.8%) can dramatically decrease smell and discharge from the tumour surface with minimal side-effects.

Necrotic tumours have a tendency to bleed and haemorrhage can be life-threatening. Caregivers should be warned of the possibility of a fatal haemorrhage and given clear instructions. Sedation with a rapidly active benzodiazepine, with or without morphine, is the most appropriate management. Dark towels could conceal the amount of blood being lost and the aim of such management is to render the patient sedated and unaware of the fatal haemorrhage.[14] Slower haemorrhage may require a vaginal packing with gauze to stop the bleeding. Longer term care may include a radiotherapy boost on the bleeding site, or embolization under radiological guidance of the arterial site causing the bleed. Patients are often anaemic, because of the chronic bleeding of advanced disease, and the use of palliative chemotherapy. In addition to blood transfusions during the acute event, iron replacement may be essential, and should be administered with erythropoietin, when indicated, to avert chronic fatigue.

Distant failure

Distant failure occurs in about 50% of patients who recur. The most common pathway for distant spread of squamous cell carcinoma is through the lymphatic system, which brings cells in the blood circulation through the thoracic duct. Once the cells enter the blood circulation, the most common metastatic pattern is lung metastases. Peritoneal seeding may occur in 20–30% of patients with distant metastatic disease and may be associated with ascites, abdominal pain and cramping, and bowel occlusion. Adenocarcinoma may cause more widespread metastatic disease, and liver involvement is not uncommon.

Lymphatic spread

The most common presentation is the appearance of a cervical or supraclavicular palpable lymph node. A thorough metastatic work-up should be done to rule other sites of tumoural spread. The mediastinum should be especially looked at, as cells must migrate through the lymphatic chains to reach the cervical anatomical area. In cases of an isolated lymph node, consideration should be given to achieving a local complete remission. Removing the affected node, if it is greater than 3 cm, followed by chemoradiation treatment, could accomplish this, although this therapeutic approach has not been systematically studied, a few patients may obtain a long-term remission.[15]

Metastases in visceral organs

Isolated metastasis An isolated metastasis should be treated with curative intent, even though most patients will suffer recurrence. If it is small (below 3 cm), a chemoradiation approach may be used. If it is bigger than 3 cm, the lesion should be resected first as radiotherapy is unlikely to eradicate all cancer cells and then treated as outlined in the isolated lymph node metastasis case above.

If the lesion is unresectable due to location or size, it should be approached with neoadjuvant chemotherapy tentatively followed by surgical resection. Chemotherapy combinations have been shown to induce more remission than single agent;[16] therefore, neoadjuvant chemotherapy should use a combination regimen. The primary goal of the neoadjuvant chemotherapy is to shrink the lesion enough that it would become resectable and a few patients may be cured with this approach.

Multiple metastases Patients with multiple metastases are usually not curable and are candidates for either a clinical trial or chemotherapy. Because chemotherapy is palliative and not curative, a clinical trial would be preferable as more knowledge may be gained on how to improve the treatment of cervical cancer. The risks and possible benefits to the patient must be clearly discussed.

If the patient is not a candidate for clinical trials, minimizing morbidity with palliative single-agent chemotherapy is preferred to multiagent treatment protocols, which offer no survival advantage. Response rates to single agents vary from 15 to 30% and complete responses are rare. The preferred drug is cisplatin (50–75 mg/m^2) or carboplatin (AUC of 6–7.5). Randomized studies of combination chemotherapy have not shown a survival advantage compared to treatment with a single agent (Table 1.1).[10] The most recent prospective comparison of single agent versus combination is a GOG study randomizing cisplatin to the combination of cisplatin and paclitaxel, which confirm the lack of survival advantage for the combination. However, cisplatin combined with paclitaxel is superior to single agent cisplatin in terms of response rate and disease free interval, at the expense of significantly higher reversible bone marrow toxicity. A comparative assessment of health-related quality of life during systemic chemotherapy of both regimens is ongoing.

In patients with squamous cell carcinoma whose disease does not respond to platinum-based chemotherapy, the only drug that has shown consistent efficacy is irinotecan.[17] This agent has been tested in five trials as a single agent in cervical cancer patients refractory to platinum-based therapy (Table 1.2). Different dosing schedules have been studied including 100 mg/m^2/week for four weeks every six weeks or for three weeks every four weeks; 150 mg/m^2 every two weeks; or 350 mg/m^2 every three weeks. The response rate varies from 13 to 26% with a median time to response of 6 weeks and a response duration of 12 weeks. The major dose-limiting side effects were nausea and vomiting (45%), diarrhea (24%), and myelosuppression (36%). Myelosuppression did not decrease when the irinotecan dose was reduced, whereas gastro-intestinal side-effects did. In the study reported by the EORTC, patients were stratified according to whether measurable disease was present outside (group A) or within (group B) the previously radiated area. Irinotecan 350 mg/m^2 was administered every three weeks. Responses occurred in 5 of 21 (24%) group A patients and in no group B patients ($n = 13$), for an overall response rate of 15%. In one study of irinotecan in patients with recurrent cervical cancer, no responses were observed. However, the authors reported that a few patients had subjective improvement and that further exploration of this drug was warranted for the treatment of cervical cancer.

For patients with adenocarcinoma not responding to platinum-based therapy, paclitaxel is currently the drug of choice as an infusion of 135–200 mg/m^2 over 24-h.[18]

Table 1.1 Randomized study of single agent cisplatin versus cisplatin-based combinations for the treatment of recurrent cervical cancer

Drugs	No Pts	CR n(%)	PR n(%)	CR + PR n(%)	Median survival (Months)	References
MMC/VCR/BLM/CDDP	54	4(7)	8(15)	12(22)	6.9	(23)
vs						
MMC/CDDP	51	2(4)	11(21)	13(25)	7.0	
vs						
CDDP	9	1(11)	2(22)	3(33)	17.0	
DBD/CDDP	438 evaluable			Same as CDDP		(24)
vs						
IFOS/CDDP				(31)	4.6	
vs						
CDDP				(18)	3.2	
BLM/VDS/MMC/CDDP	201 evaluable	(11)	(31)	(42)	10.1	(25)
vs						
CDDP		(7)	(18)	(25)	9.3	

MMC, Mitomycin C; VCR, Vincristine; BLM, Bleomycin; CDDP < Cisplatin; DBD, Dibromodulcitol; IFOS, Ifosfamide; VDS, Vindesine.

Table 1.2 Trials of irinotecan in cervical cancer[17]

Dose	Schedule	No Patients	CR	PR	OR
125 mg/m^2	Weekly × 4	42	2% (1)	19% (8)	21% (9)
125 mg/m^2	Weekly × 4	45	2% (1)	11% (5)	13% (6)
350 mg/m^2	q 3 weeks				
	group A	21	5% (1)	19% (4)	24% (5)
	group B	13	0% (0)	0% (0)	0% (0)
100 mg/m^2	Weekly × 4	24	8% (2)	13% (3)	21% (5)
150 mg/m^2	q 2 weeks × 3	31	10% (3)	16% (5)	26% (8)
Total		176	4% (8)	14% (25)	19% (33)

CR = complete response; PR = partial response.

Peritoneal metastases

Patients should receive primary chemotherapy for the recurrent peritoneal disease as outlined in the paragraph on distant metastases. Intraperitoneal chemotherapy has not been studied in patients with peritoneal metastases of cervical cancer. Though less frequent than other patterns of metastatic spread, peritoneal spread can pose a therapeutic challenge, as the symptomatology is similar to patients affected with stage III ovarian cancer. Symptoms include nausea, vomiting, constipation, ascites, and bowel obstruction. Appropriate radiographic evaluation is important, to select the patient likely to benefit from resection, bypass, or diversion. Patients with generalized carcinomatosis are unlikely to benefit from surgical intervention. Nutrition may become a daily problem, generally distressing the family.

Treatment of complications

The management of bowel dysfunction or obstruction, and ascites, common manifestations of distant recurrence, has been discussed in separate Chapters 7 and 10.

Nutrition Anxiety over nutrition is very common in caregivers of patients with terminal diseases. Special foods, such as enteric and parenteral feedings, may be associated with high cost, potential complications and complex ethical issues. Megestrol acetate has been used as an appetite stimulant in cancer cachexia, but is expensive. Metoclopramide has a gastrokinetic effect that could be beneficial. Creative gastronomy with nutritious soups and drinks can do much to improve food intake; however, forcing food in a dying patient is not appropriate. Family members need to be told, in an emotionally supportive way, that their relative now has less desire and need for food. Total parenteral nutrition and intravenous hydration have not been shown to benefit dying patients.[19]

Emotional support

Emotional support is crucial to the well-being of suffering patients. Distress has more than just a physical origin, and may be due to lack of stable emotional support, fragile social and financial conditions, or spiritual anguish (Fig. 1.6). Depression occurs in at least 20% of cancer patients and is often under-treated. Patient's fear of the future, feelings of guilt, unresolved anger and grief need to be elicited, and discussed with her. Outcomes need to be discussed with the caregiver, the immediate family, and the children.

Questions about the meaning of life and death are deep spiritual questions transcending the practice of a formal religion. An atmosphere of trust and acceptance, with honest communication, is essential for the distressed patient to express her deepest concerns and to accept the progression of the disease. The spiritual dimension of the individual patient should always be respected. Chaplaincy services may provide significant support to patients and families who need or desire to confide their vulnerability.[20]

Advance directives and a durable power of attorney will allow a competent patient to express their wishes for later medical management when they become unable to give informed consent. It is an integral part of the medical interaction between patient and physician. Written records should be kept to document the patient's wishes. Arrangements for the care of surviving children should be recommended, and a will needs to be properly drawn to settle any pending affairs or unfinished business.

It is very important to maintain the patient's dignity during the dying process, especially when patients are not able to take care of themselves. The caring focus has to be on comfort and symptom control more than therapeutic

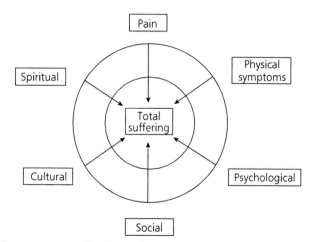

Fig. 1.6 The components of suffering. (With permission.)

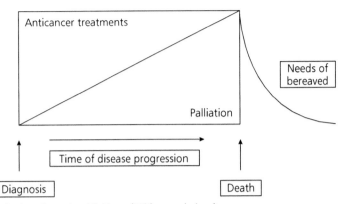

Fig. 1.7 Patients' needs with time. (With permission.)

interventions (Fig. 1.7). Consultation with a palliative care team should take place early enough in the disease process. The family must be allowed to grieve at the bedside. A calm and peaceful death appears to contribute to relatives' ability to cope in bereavement. Children often blame themselves for the death of a parent and should not be excluded from their dying mother.[21] It may be the only time they will have to remember their mother in a constructive way, and participation in the dying process may avoid guilt feelings in the future. The creation of a treasure chest will give them tangible memories of their mother. There are books available to help adults communicating with children and answering their questions.

The social hardship that is associated with loss of the family structure and of income may only have an impact on the family after the funeral. A condolence letter with an invitation to answer questions can be very supportive to the mourning family.[22]

References

1 Sherris, J., Herdman C., and Elias, C. (2001). Cervical cancer in the developing world. *Western Journal of Medicine*, 175(4): 231–233.

2 Jemal, A., Thomas, A., Murray, T., and Thun, M. (2002). Cancer statistics, 2002. *Cancer Journal for Clinicians*, 52(1): 23–47.

3 Schoell, W. M., Janicek, M. F., and Mirhashemi, R. (1999). Epidemiology and biology of cervical cancer. [Review] [42 refs]. *Seminars in Surgical Oncology*, 16(3): 203–211.

4 Eifel, P., Berek, J., and Thigpen, J. (2001). Cancer of the cervix, vagina and vulva. In *Cancer: Principles and Practice of Oncology* (ed. V. DeVita, S. Hellman, and S. Rosenberg), p. 1547. Lippincott: Philadelphia.

5 Thomas, G. M. (1999). Improved treatment for cervical cancer–concurrent chemotherapy and radiotherapy. *New Eng J Med*, 340(15): 1198–1200.

6 Bergmark, K., Avall-Lundqvist, E., Dickman, P. W., Henningsohn, L., and Steineck, G. (1999). Vaginal changes and sexuality in women with a history of cervical cancer. *New Eng J Med*, 340(18): 1383–1389.

7 Zeisler, H., Joura, E. A., Moeschl, P., Maier, U., and Koelbl, H. (1997). Preoperative evaluation of tumour extension in patients with recurrent cervical cancer. *Acta Obstetricia et Gynecologica Scandinavica*, 76(5): 474–477.

8 Shepherd, J. H., Crawford, R. A., Christmas, T. J., and Hendry, W. F. (1997). Total pelvic reconstruction after exenteration for recurrent cervical cancer. *Br J Urology*, 80 (Suppl 1): 79–81.

9 Sommers, G. M., Grigsby, P. W., Perez, C. A., Camel, H. M., Kao, M. S., Galakatos, A. E. *et al.* (1989). Outcome of recurrent cervical carcinoma following definitive irradiation. *Gynecol Oncol*, 35(2): 150–155.

10 Nguyen, H. N. and Nordqvist, S. R. (1999). Chemotherapy of advanced and recurrent cervical carcinoma. *Semin Surg Oncol*, 16(3): 247–250.

11 Emmert, C. and Kohler, U. (1996). Management of genital fistulas in patients with cervical cancer. *Arch GynecolObstet*, 259(1): 19–24.

12 Harrington, K. J., Pandha, H. S., Kelly, S. A., Lambert, H. E., Jackson, J. E., and Waxman, J. (1995). Palliation of obstructive nephropathy due to malignancy. *Brit J Urol*, 76(1): 101–107.

13 Smith, C. (1995). Alterations of untreated lympho-oedema and its grades over time. *Lymphology*, 28: 174–185.

14 Finlay, I. (1998). Management of the dying patient. In *Principles and Practice of Geriatric Medicine*, p. 1467–1477.

15 Sakurai, H., Mitsuhashi, N., Takahashi, M., Akimoto, T., Muramatsu, H. Ishikawa, H. *et al.* (2001). Analysis of recurrence of squamous cell carcinoma of the uterine cervix after definitive radiation therapy alone: patterns of recurrence, latent periods, and prognosis. *Internat J Radiation Oncol, Biol, Phys*, 50(5): 1136–1144.

16 Kumar, L., Pokharel, Y. H., Kumar, S., Singh, R., Rath, G. K., and Kochupillai, V. (1998). Single agent versus combination chemotherapy in recurrent cervical cancer. *J Obstet Gynaecol Res*, 24(6): 401–409.

17 Verschraegen, C. (2002). Irinotecan for the treatment of cervical cancer. *Oncol* (Huntington), 16(5 Suppl 5): 32–34.

18 Curtin, J. P., Blessing, J. A., Webster, K. D., Rose, P. G., Mayer, A. R., Fowler, Jr., W. C. *et al.* (2001). Paclitaxel, an active agent in nonsquamous carcinomas of the uterine cervix: a Gynecologic Oncology Group Study. *J Clin Oncol*, 19(5): 1275–1278.

19 Ellershaw, J., Sutcliffe, J., and Saunders, C. (1995). Dehydration and the dying patient. *J Pain Symp Manage*, 10: 192–197.

20 Hilliard, N. (1998). Spirituality in hospice care. *Palliative Care Today*, 6(4): 52–53.

21 Black, D. (1998). Coping with loss: bereavement in childhood, *Br Med J*, 316: 931–933.

22 Lerner, A. (2001). Letters of condolence, *New Eng J Med*, 345(5): 374.

23 Alberts, D. S., Kronmal, R., Baker, L. H., Stock-Novack, D. L., Surwit, E. A., Boutselis, J. G. *et al.* (1987). Phase II randomized trial of cisplatin chemotherapy regimens in the treatment of recurrent or metastatic squamous cell cancer of the cervix: a Southwest Oncology Group Study. *J Clin Oncol*, 5(11): 1791–1795.

24 Omura, G.A., Blessing, J. A., Vaccarello, L., Berman, M. L., Clarke-Pearson, D. L., Mutch, D. G. *et al.* (1997). Randomized trial of cisplatin versus cisplatin plus mitolactol versus cisplatin plus ifosfamide in advanced squamous carcinoma of the cervix: a Gynecologic Oncology Group study. *J Clin Oncol*, 15(1): 165–171.

25 Vermorken, J.B., Zanetta, G., De Oliveira, C. F., van der Burg, M. E., Lacave, A. J., Teodorovic, I. *et al.* (2001). Randomized phase III trial of bleomycin, vindesine, mitomycin-C, and cisplatin (BEMP) versus cisplatin (P) in disseminated squamous-cell carcinoma of the uterine cervix: an EORTC Gynecological Cancer Cooperative Group study. *Ann Oncol*, 12(7): 967–974.

Chapter 2

The assessment and management of advanced cancer of the ovary

Bristi Basu, Cheryl Palmer, Jean Abraham, and Helena Earl

Introduction

Ovarian cancer is the seventh most common cancer of women worldwide and is responsible for the highest mortality rates from gynaecological malignancy in North America and Europe. Although ovarian cancer is generally regarded as a chemo-sensitive malignancy, the majority of women will ultimately develop chemo-resistance, and die of their disease. Only 15–20% of women presenting with poor-risk ovarian cancer (stage IIIc and IV) are curable with a combination of chemotherapy and surgery. At first presentation, therefore, the oncologist and gynae-oncology surgeon, will offer as intensive chemotherapy as is tolerable, and also at some point carry out surgery to remove as much of the tumour as possible.

However, when women relapse there is *no* prospect of cure and the aims of treatment change to palliation of symptoms and prolongation of life. When cancers remain sensitive to chemotherapy, this may be the best way to palliate symptoms of disease. Some women with ovarian cancer may have long periods of time living with metastatic disease, receiving intermittent courses of chemotherapy. The management of these patients, who are incurable but remain sensitive to chemotherapy, becomes a complex balancing act. This involves trying to judge likely response rates and side-effects of chemotherapy in different individuals, with different cancers, and different attitudes to their disease and to life in general. The aims of management can be summarized in a phrase often used in our clinics: 'we want to keep you as well as possible for as long as possible'. This conveys to the patient the aspects of caring and 'aiming to do our best', which are so important; the notion that chemotherapy is likely to prolong their lives; but also communicates the complexity of decision-making: 'we hope to prolong your life but we don't want you to pay too high a price in terms of toxicity'. However, we must be clear that the only judge of what is 'too much', is the patient herself.

Our view is that most patients (although not all) welcome the opportunity to hand over (although not completely) these difficult decisions to someone they 'trust'. I think this point is well illustrated by Dr Ingelfinger's narrative of his own diagnosis of oesophageal cancer.[1] As the editor of the *New England Journal of Medicine* he was not short of advice about how his cancer should be managed, but he longed for a kind, compassionate, experienced doctor to come along and make the best decisions with him and for him. I would see one of our most important functions as oncologists involved in the 'active' management of ovarian cancer, to lead patients to make the best decisions about their active treatment. The 'active palliative' management (and this is *not* an oxymoron) of women with advanced ovarian cancer requires an essentially close relationship between the oncology team and the palliative care team in hospital practice, and the primary care based and community specialist palliative care team at home. In best ovarian cancer management it is important that we all have a real understanding of what the 'other' team has to offer (oncology for the palliative care team and vice versa), and this understanding will make an important difference to the lives of women with advanced ovarian cancer, which is what this is all about.

Aims of chapter

This chapter will highlight some of the evidence base for treatment decisions facing oncologists in the management of women with ovarian cancer presenting with advanced or recurrent disease. Emphasis will be placed on the role of chemotherapy in these settings. Aims of treatment will differ for patients based on factors such as their disease process, performance status, and co-morbid illnesses, and their individual wishes. Three case histories have been included to highlight some of these clinical scenarios and different management decisions.

Sources for this chapter

Sources of evidence for this chapter included a search of Medline for key review articles in the English language, and more recently published phase II and phase III trial data. Information from the Advanced Ovarian Cancer Trialists Group is included as updated in the Cochrane Review for chemotherapy for advanced ovarian cancer. Lastly personal experience from our centre has been included in the form of three individual case histories in which management was shared with the hospital-based palliative care team.

Diagnosis and staging

The European Organisation for Research and Treatment of Cancer (EORTC) and the American Society of Clinical Oncology (ASCO) recommend that all women fit for surgery, regardless of clinical stage, should undergo a full staging laparotomy with ascitic fluid sampling for cytology and review of retroperitoneal and pelvic lymph nodes. This is to acquire accurate information on disease stage using the International Federation of Gynaecology and Obstetrics (FIGO) classification. The FIGO stage can provide prognostic information and be used to separate patients into different groups: those having early and those having advanced disease at presentation (Table 2.1). Advanced disease is stage II and beyond, with evidence of macroscopic spread

Table 2.1 Epithelial ovarian cancer – TNM Clinical Classification and International Federation of Gynaecology and Obstetrics (FIGO) staging system

TNM category	FIGO stages	Characteristics
Tx		Primary tumour cannot be assessed
T0		No evidence of primary tumour
T1	I	Tumour limited to the ovaries
T1a	IA	Tumour limited to one ovary, capsule intact, no tumour on ovarian surface; no malignant cells in ascites or peritoneal washings
T1b	IB	Tumour limited to both ovaries; capsule intact, no tumour on ovarian surface; no malignant cells in ascites or peritoneal washings
T1c	IC	Tumour limited to one or both ovaries with any of the following: capsule ruptured, tumour on ovarian surface, malignant cells in ascites or peritoneal washings
T2	II	Tumour involves one or both ovaries with pelvic extension
T2a	IIA	Extension and/or implants on uterus and/or tubes; no malignant cells in ascites or peritoneal washings
T2b	IIB	Extension to other pelvic tissues; no malignant cells in ascites or peritoneal washings
T2c	IIC	Pelvic extension with malignant cells in ascites or peritoneal washings
T3 and/or N1	III	Tumour involves one or both ovaries with microscopically confirmed peritoneal metastasis outside the pelvis and/or regional lymph node metastasis
T3a	IIIA	Microscopic peritoneal metastasis beyond pelvis
T3b	IIIB	Macroscopic peritoneal metastasis beyond pelvis 2 cm or less in greatest dimension
T3C and/or N1	IIIC	Peritoneal metastasis beyond pelvis more than 2 cm in greatest dimension and/or regional lymph node metastasis
M1	IV	Distant metastasis (excludes peritoneal metastasis)

Note: liver capsule metastasis is T3/Stage III, liver parenchymal metastasis M1/Stage IV. Pleural effusion must have positive cytology for M1/Stage IV outside the ovaries. Even within the advanced group there is a range of outcomes from women who have short prognoses to those who are cured of their disease. Treatment aims will therefore have to take into account this range when assessing the individual patient's risk versus benefit.

Treatment for advanced disease at initial presentation

Ovarian cancer spreads early in the disease process into the abdominal cavity from the pelvis. Often advanced disease will manifest as large pelvic masses at surgery with further lesions involving the peritoneum covering the bowel, mesentery, omentum, and liver. Standard treatment of advanced disease combines a multimodality approach with cytoreductive surgery and combination chemotherapy using platinum/taxane drugs. Ovarian cancer is a highly chemotherapy-sensitive malignancy. With current treatment the majority of patients presenting with advanced disease will show an objective response with a significant, sustained improvement in cancer-related symptoms. Unfortunately most women will eventually relapse and will need to be considered for second-line treatment.

Surgery

Standard surgical treatment for women with advanced ovarian cancer is surgical staging and attempted debulking surgery to remove as much tumour as possible, soon after diagnosis and prior to any chemotherapy. This 'standard' management has evolved over time, and is largely predicated on women being referred to the surgeon first. Given that ovarian cancer is advanced in the majority of women at presentation, radical surgery is an unusual first approach and is different from the standard in other cancers, e.g. colorectal cancer metastatic to the liver and abdominal cavity. However as the practice evolved further through time, surgeons defined what appear to be important prognostic groupings depending on how much of the metastatic tumour was removed. The size of residual disease after surgery is one of the most important prognostic factors for survival. Patients with resection of all macroscopic disease are classed as having optimal cytoreduction and have a 2-year survival of 80% in contrast with less than 22% in patients with lesions larger than 2 cm.[2] There has been much discussion about what this really means: is the improved prognosis only a result of the expertise of the specialist surgeon, or partly an inherent tumour characteristic, which not only gives the patient a better prognosis but also makes the tumour easier to remove. 'Post hoc' rationalization of these surgical findings include the possibility that successful surgical debulking down to tumour nodules <2 cm improves response rates to chemotherapy by removing tumour tissue, which is already resistant to chemotherapy, and improving chemotherapy delivery to the smaller residual nodules of tumour. Although there is some experimental *in vitro* evidence for this, there is no randomized clinical evidence.

When primary surgery is technically difficult or impossible, and/or the patient is unfit at the time of diagnosis to undergo a radical surgical procedure, then chemotherapy can be given prior to interval debulking surgery. There is evidence from a randomized trial carried out by the EORTC that interval-debulking surgery improves disease-free and overall survival in this poor prognosis group.[3] All patients, including those with unfavourable prognostic factors such as stage IV disease, widespread peritoneal disease, or ascites at primary surgery, seem to benefit from interval cytoreduction, showing an increase in progression-free survival and overall survival. Interval debulking is offered also to patients with stable disease after primary chemotherapy.

Chemotherapy

Ovarian cancer can be considered a 'chemo-sensitive' solid epithelial malignancy. This is important in the palliative context because it means that patients may go on responding to chemotherapy for some years with significant treatment-free intervals and good quality of life between courses of chemotherapy. What does 'chemo-sensitive' mean? Ovarian cancer will respond with either a partial or complete response in 70–85% of patients given first-line therapy. Response is assessed clinically, by measuring tumour masses and also the resolution of ascites (a common problem in ovarian cancer); radiologically using ultrasound or CT scans; and serologically using the Ca-125 serum marker of ovarian cancer. This marker is present in the blood of about 85% of women with ovarian cancer, and if positive is a very useful marker to monitor response to chemotherapy. Metastatic disease in the peritoneum is difficult to visualize, particularly when the size of individual tumour nodules is small. However Gynae-oncology Centres, where all ovarian cancer patients are assessed at the time of diagnosis, have expert radiologists skilled at documenting small volume peritoneal disease. Computerized tomography (CT) technology is improving rapidly and with higher resolution, more detailed CT imaging, will come an increased ability to define small-volume disease. The response category of 'partial response' means that the radiologically and serologically defined disease has decreased by at least half of that seen at the start of therapy. The meaning of the 'complete response' category is obvious. In ovarian cancer, response will significantly reduce tumour symptoms of pain, discomfort, sub-acute intestinal obstruction, and the re-accumulation of ascites. Therefore a high rate of objective response will bring a high rate of symptom control. General symptoms of advanced cancer, i.e. poor appetite, weight loss, low albumin and leg oedema, poor nutritional status, muscle wasting, and thrombosis, will also gradually improve if the patient responds to treatment. When ovarian cancer continues to respond to second- and third-line therapies, patients have a maintained good quality of life.

Role of platinum agents

Cisplatin gained a definite place in the primary treatment of ovarian cancer some years ago. More recently single-agent carboplatin has been shown to be equivalent to cisplatin/cyclosphamide/adriamycin (CAP) in the ICON 2 study and is much less toxic.

Role of paclitaxel first-line with carboplatin

The International Collaborative Ovarian Neoplasm (ICON) Group recently reported the ICON 3 study.[4] This compared paclitaxel plus carboplatin versus standard chemotherapy with either single-agent carboplatin or CAP, in women with ovarian cancer. This study raises some interesting and important questions for the ovarian cancer research community in the UK, and perhaps most importantly for women suffering with advanced ovarian cancer. This study did not confirm an advantage for ovarian cancer patients from the addition of paclitaxel, despite two other studies that produced a strongly positive result. We feel it is important for readers to have a full understanding of the place of these therapies in the treatment of women with advanced and relapsed ovarian cancer and therefore will take some time to discuss this result further.

There are already two large trials, GOG 111 (410 patients)[5] and the Inter-group Study OV10 (680 patients),[6] which show median survival advantages of 14 and 10 months, respectively (highly statistically significant) for the addition of paclitaxel to platinum as first-line therapy. GOG 111 entry was restricted to patients with high-risk stage III and IV disease who had been sub-optimally debulked. OV10 did include some high-risk stage II patients, but neither study included the early stage lower risk patients who were part of ICON 3. If the analysis of outcome in ICON 3 is restricted to stage III and IV patients with >2 cm residual bulk disease (i.e. a similar patient group to GOG 111), then there emerges a difference in favour of the paclitaxel/carboplatin combination (although not quite statistically significant). However, combined with GOG 111 and OV10 results, ICON 3 will contribute evidence for the benefit of paclitaxel with carboplatin first-line in this poor risk group.

In Europe we might criticize US gynaecological oncologists, for almost immediately extending the indications for platinum/paclitaxel chemotherapy to early stage, low-risk patients following publication of the GOG 111 results in January 1996. By the same token we will be justly criticized by the rest of the world if we deny our high-risk stage III and IV ovarian cancer patients combined first-line therapy on account of the ICON 3 data. Given our aims in the UK to deliver improvements in cancer survival rates to approach outcomes already achieved in the rest of continental Europe by 2005, it would be a truly backward step to withdraw treatment proven to be effective, from the ovarian cancer group with the worst prognosis.

We have commenced a phase I/II randomized translational study in Cambridge, in which we utilize delayed surgery in women with stage IIIc–IV disease, to give monotherapy (either carboplatin or paclitaxel) prior to surgery.[7] This study looks at prospective molecular profiling and candidate gene expression as predictors of response and resistance to carboplatin and paclitaxel given as monotherapy. Window studies like this will increase our ability to individualize therapy by defining robust, predictive molecular profiles of response to different treatments.

Duration of treatment

The duration of first-line chemotherapy is usually six cycles, although if the patient has residual disease and is continuing to respond, therapy may be extended to nine cycles. In second- and third-line therapy we would usually limit therapy to six cycles. When there is no prospect of cure, therapy should be given for as short a time as possible to induce a useful remission.

Dose intensification

It is unproven whether dose intensity is more important than total dose delivered in the treatment of ovarian cancer. It must always be borne in mind that for the majority of women with advanced ovarian disease, the treatment is palliative making quality of life an important issue. There is an ongoing European study of high-dose chemotherapy in women who have been maximally debulked, and have no residual disease at the completion of primary therapy. There is little data yet on the effectiveness of this in ovarian cancer and it is not a strategy that has proved effective in other common solid tumours, e.g. breast cancer.

Intraperitoneal chemotherapy

Intraperitoneal administration of chemotherapy agents has been suggested as a technique to improve the efficacy of therapy of malignant disease principally confined to the peritoneal cavity. Data from phase I studies suggest safety and pharmacokinetic advantage for intraperitoneal drug delivery, with responses being shown in the phase II trial setting. Randomized phase III studies have also shown a survival benefit associated with administration of intraperitoneal cisplatin compared to intravenous chemotherapy when used as initial treatment of small volume residual advanced ovarian cancer.[8]

Relapsed disease

Ovarian cancer usually presents as advanced disease, which often remains confined to the peritoneal cavity. Recent *in vitro* studies growing ovarian cancer cells in culture showed that in the pH of the peritoneal cavity (which is significantly lower that the normal physiological pH of 7.4), ovarian cancer cells proliferate by activating growth factors and growth factor receptors. However, at normal body pH the ovarian cancer cells become quiescent. This may be one explanation of the extra-ordinary clinical pattern of spread of ovarian cancer, with disease remaining largely in the peritoneal and pleural cavities. Although ovarian cancer can spread into the liver, lungs, bones, and brain, this happens rarely and often only very late in the disease.

Despite surgical cytoreduction and first-line chemotherapy, the majority of advanced ovarian cancer patients will require second-line treatment for recurrent disease. Disease relapse after primary treatment occurs in over 60% of ovarian cancer patients overall, and in over 80% of patients who are diagnosed initially with advanced disease. Median time to progression is less than two years.

Surgery for relapsed ovarian cancer

Second debulking procedures at relapse have limited benefit for patients and there have been no randomized trials addressing this question. In our practice the only time we would consider this is when there has been >5 years from primary diagnosis, and when debulking surgery can be easily achieved.

The pattern of spread of ovarian cancer to peritoneal and pleural surfaces commonly produces widespread disease over the small bowel, omentum, and mesentery. This produces 'sub-acute intestinal obstruction', which is so commonly seen in ovarian cancer. Surgery in general is not helpful to manage this, and we will leave other contributors in this book to discuss medical management of sub-acute obstruction. Occasionally a large tumour mass can produce an acute obstruction that can be helped by surgical intervention, or there may be two or three major sites of obstruction that can be helped with by-pass surgery (see Case 2), but in this phase of the illness surgery will more often be harmful and hasten death. These are difficult decisions, which must be made by close liaison between the surgical, non-surgical, and palliative care teams. The development of Gynae-oncology Centres has provided for the evolution of a group of people who are making these difficult decisions repeatedly, so the co-ordinated management of these patients has been much improved in recent years.

Chemotherapy in relapsed ovarian cancer

Significance of platinum-free interval

Treatment planning is based around the concept of platinum sensitivity, or the platinum-free interval. Thus women whose disease progresses whilst on platinum therapy are classified as having platinum-refractory disease. If they relapse within 6 months of receiving platinum, they have platinum-resistant disease. Patients are classed as having platinum-sensitive disease if they relapse after 6 months.

The probability of response to second-line chemotherapy following platinum-based treatments is related to the platinum-free interval. Other factors shown to have some predictive value include tumour burden and histology. Salvage monochemotherapy is generally used, but when the platinum-free interval is longer than 24 months, re-treatment with platinum compounds and/or taxanes is indicated. The response rates seen when the treatment-free interval exceeds 24 months are almost equivalent to that of primary chemotherapy.[9]

Patients with platinum-refractory or platinum-resistant disease are encouraged to enter clinical trials of therapy, which often include non-platinum agents. A number of new agents have demonstrated activity in ovarian cancer. These drugs include liposomal doxorubicin (Caelyx), gemcitabine, and topotecan.

Treatment beyond second line

There are many and increasing numbers of chemotherapy treatments for ovarian cancer that can be used at relapse. As referred to above, if the treatment-free interval is >12 months then there is nearly a 50% chance that single-agent carboplatin will remain effective. In patients with a long treatment-free interval this is therefore the treatment of choice.

Recently Van der Burg et al. published the results of their study from the Netherlands on intensive cisplatin and etoposide therapy in relapsed ovarian cancer patients.[10] The study included 170 patients who were treated with induction therapy of cisplatin 50 or 70 mg/m^2 on days 1, 8, 15, 29, 36, and 43, in conjunction with oral etoposide 50 mg daily for days 1–15 and 29–43. Those patients with response or stable disease were then placed on maintenance therapy with oral etoposide for 21 days in 28 for a further six to nine cycles. Weekly chemotherapy administration has been used in treatment of other solid tumours, in an attempt to modify the toxicity profile whilst maintaining efficacy. Weekly epirubicin is used in metastatic breast cancer patients who have bone marrow infiltration, or who are frail, as it is seen to produce less myelotoxicity and is generally well tolerated. The rationale behind the Van der Burg study, however, was to intensify the dose delivery of cisplatin to induce remission and to follow this with maintenance oral chemotherapy, to keep the established remission for as long as possible.

Thirty-eight patients assessed had 'platinum-sensitive' disease, of whom 92% showed a response, with median survival of 26 months. The 'platinum-intermediate' disease group (platinum-free interval of 4–12 months) showed 91% of patients responding, with median survival of 16 months. Of most interest, however, was the response seen in the group termed 'platinum-refractory'. This group included 28 patients, of whom 46% responded, although this response was short-lived, with median duration of five months and median survival of 13 months.

Toxicity reported in the much-publicized paper in January 2002, included myelotoxicity, although only 10% of patients required a delay in treatment of more than one week. Reported non-haematological toxicity was relatively uncommon, with nephrotoxicity in 4%, and grade II sensory neuropathy in only 7% of patients.

These excellent second-line response rates and low rates of toxicity persuaded us to give this treatment to some of our patients, and indeed many of them had read about this treatment in newspapers and were keen to try it. Unfortunately, although we have seen some good radiological and serological responses with the treatment, many have experienced severe side-effects, with marked reduction in general performance status during treatment, loss of appetite and taste, severe fatigue, nephrotoxicity resulting in profound and prolonged hypomagnesaemia, and grade II–III peripheral sensory neuropathy. Indeed, we have had one treatment-related death from neutropenic sepsis. Our view is that patient selection is of prime importance when offering such intensive treatment (see Case 3). For the majority of women with relapsed ovarian cancer, this therapy is too toxic whatever the potential gain, because after all it will not ultimately cure patients.

Other potential second-line therapies include paclitaxel, topotecan, liposomal doxorubicin, oxaliplatin, irinotecan, and gemcitabine. Combinations of cisplatin, epirubicin, and continuous 5-fluouracil (5FU) have been used extensively.

Oral chemotherapy

The oldest oral agent available to these patients is chlorambucil, which can still be used to good effect in some of our patients who have already had multiple lines of previous chemotherapy (see Case 2). The development of oral 5FU equivalents (capecitabine and uftoral) will probably see these oral agents replace continuous intravenous infusion 5FU, as they avoid the infection and thrombosis risks, which accompany the insertion of Hickman lines in these patients. Other oral agents include etoposide as used in the Van der Burg regimen. This has very variable oral bio availability (ranging from 30 to 90%), and this coupled with high drug–albumin binding, make the side-effects (particularly myelosuppression and mucositis) difficult to predict. Women with advanced or recurrent ovarian cancer frequently have low serum albumin levels, and as protein binding of etoposide is most dependent on serum albumin levels, this means that levels of free and active etoposide are higher in these women and cause severe toxicity.[11]

Ultimately the true aim of salvage chemotherapy in relapsed ovarian cancer remains palliative, as cure is not possible, complete responses are rare, and responses are seldom long-lasting. The main objectives of salvage chemotherapy will include improvement in quality of life and symptoms, tumour load reduction, and survival advantage. Response rate (range from 15 to 50%) and response duration to different single agents are similar, therefore patient convenience, toxicities from previous treatment, side-effects, and cost are all factors in deciding on the salvage chemotherapy regimen to be administered.

Biological therapies and immunotherapy

There is currently much clinical development of biological approaches to the treatment of patients with ovarian cancer. Drugs being tested include those interfering with angiogenic processes, signal transduction pathways, and matrix metalloproteinase function. Future directions for treatment of ovarian cancer may include a new concept of treatment in which patients receive polychemotherapy together with a biological agent, followed by chronic maintenance treatment with biological therapy.

Immunotherapy techniques are also under investigation for treatment of recurrence. These include antitumour monoclonal antibodies. Antibodies to ovarian cancer antigen have also been combined with radioisotopes, immuno-toxins, and chemotherapeutic drug conjugates to improve targeting. Other methods include vaccines designed to excite cellular and humoral immune responses against ovarian cancer, and modification of antigen-presenting cells to stimulate antitumour immune response.

Quality of life assessments and patients' expectations

Quality of life is an important part of all cancer therapy, none more than in ovarian cancer. In patients with recurrent or refractory ovarian cancer, the aims of treating with chemotherapy are palliation of disease-related symptoms, with improvement in quality and, to some extent, length of life. In many ovarian cancer trials much information is collected on toxicity of chemotherapy and general quality of life using Common Toxicity Criteria (CTC), which are the same across the globe, and the EORTC quality of life patient reported questionnaires for cancer patients, with the new ovarian cancer module. Although routine quality of life is not usually collected in patients outside clinical trials, there is nevertheless a constant analysis going on concerning 'pain versus gain'. An attempt is made to weigh the degree of response occurring against the toxicity that the woman is experiencing.

Many studies evaluating palliative chemotherapy in advanced ovarian cancer have relied on surrogate measures of patient benefit using biomedical responses rather than appraising palliative end-points such as quality of life and clinical benefit. This issue has been addressed in a Canadian study prospectively evaluating patient expectation, palliative outcomes of chemotherapy, and the resource utilization in patients undergoing second- or third-line chemotherapy for recurrent or refractory advanced ovarian cancer.[12] Quality of life was assessed using EORTC Quality of Life Questionnaire C30 (QLQ C30) and Functional Assessment of Cancer Therapy-Ovarian (FACT-O).

In the study, objective responses were seen in seven of 27 patients, with median survival of 11 months. Interestingly 65% of women expected that chemotherapy would make them live longer and 42% that it would cure them, suggesting that patient expectations from treatment are often unrealistic. However, after two cycles of treatment, quality of life improvement was seen, especially in global function and emotional function with EORTC QLQ C30. This improvement was sustained for a median of 2 and 3 months, respectively. Therefore, despite the fact that objective responses were low, active palliation with chemotherapy seems to be associated with improvements in patients' emotional function and global quality of life.[13]

Case histories

Case 1

This is a 53-year-old highly articulate and intelligent woman who was diagnosed with primary peritoneal adenocarcinoma in 1999. Her initial laparoscopy showed widespread disease scattered on the peritoneum and diaphragm with nodules in the pelvis and ascites. She had a pleural effusion, which was cytologically documented to be serous papillary carcinoma, conferring stage IV status to her disease. She was entered on a clinical trial (SCOTROC 1) and post-operatively received six cycles of carboplatin and paclitaxel, followed by three further cycles of single-agent carboplatin. This course of treatment resulted in grade II peripheral neurotoxicity, myalgia, mucositis, alopecia, and fatigue. Despite this, her WHO performance status was unchanged at the end of treatment at performance status 1. She remained on follow-up and had regular serum Ca-125 measurements. Eight months later she was noted to have a rising Ca-125, although she was not symptomatic. A CT scan unfortunately did confirm relapse and a long discussion ensued on the timing of further treatment. The patient was extremely well with no symptoms and was feeling a loss of autonomy regarding her medical treatment. She elected not to have her Ca-125 levels monitored further and decided her treatment should be driven more by symptoms than by biochemistry. Nine months after this she started to note pelvic pain and constipation, and following confirmation of disease progression on CT scan and rising Ca-125 levels, decided to receive chemotherapy. Given her long treatment-free interval she received single-agent carboplatin. This resulted initially in resolution of her pelvic symptoms and little toxicity. Her post-treatment scans, however, showed radiological evidence of progressive disease. She began to develop signs of this progression with abdominal pain and bloating. Further chemotherapy options were discussed, including the intensive Van der Burg cisplatin/etoposide combination and newer drugs such as liposomal doxorubicin and topotecan. The patient was referred for a formal Macmillan (specialist palliative care) review and 'end of life issues' were discussed, as well as the pros and cons of palliative care alone versus palliative care with inclusion of chemotherapy. She was made aware of the problems she may encounter as her disease progressed. Medications were started for her symptoms. The patient herself performed an Internet search and in consultation with her husband decided that she did not want any more chemotherapy. She therefore was managed symptomatically with low residue diet, laxatives, antispasmodics, and ascitic drainage when needed. She died two and a half years from diagnosis, having completed a PhD, and seen her only son through his A' level course and on to university.

An acknowledgement in her PhD thesis read:

> I also owe much to Dr Helena Earl and the her team. They are all no doubt very skilled practitioners. But best of all I was allowed to be in control of my life. Thank you.

And from her husband after her death:

> Thank you for your professionalism, your honesty, your 'hunches' and above all for allowing M to be in control.

Case 2

This is a 36-year-old woman who was diagnosed with an early stage well-differentiated ovarian carcinoma in 1999 for which she underwent initial surgery followed by single-agent carboplatin chemotherapy, as she was concerned with potential toxicities from a taxane. She unfortunately relapsed a year later with widespread peritoneal nodules noted at laparoscopy, which were confirmed to be ovarian adenocarcinoma. She elected to receive chemotherapy with carboplatin and paclitaxel, but encountered problems with nausea and vomiting on this combination. Following three cycles of treatment she underwent debulking surgery. Her disease was debulked to less than 0.5 cm. She completed a total of six cycles carboplatin and paclitaxel, and sustained some mild peripheral neurotoxicity from this. A post-treatment scan showed very little in the way of residual disease, although there was comment on some calcification at areas where previous nodules existed. On the basis of this she was offered three further cycles of single-agent carboplatin, but she was unable to tolerate more than one treatment because of severe nausea and fatigue. She declined further chemotherapy and was kept on follow-up. Almost immediately she developed symptoms of sub-acute bowel obstruction and eventually required an inpatient admission to control her symptoms. She failed to settle with symptomatic measures including hyoscine, diamorphine, and methotrimeprazine via syringe driver and addition of dexamethasone. CT scan images were consistent with mechanical obstruction with bowel loops adherent at the terminal ileum. Her case was discussed at a multidisciplinary meeting with surgical and palliative care teams, where the options were spelt out:

- percutaneous gastrostomy as a purely palliative method of venting her bowel, if she decided against major surgery;
- defunctioning ileostomy with possibility of high output via the stoma and psychological issues relating to this;
- palliative bypass of the small bowel.

She elected to have laparotomy and palliative internal bypass of the obstructed loops of bowel in the pelvis. She made a good post-operative recovery and, with dietary advice on low residue products, was able to maintain a satisfactory oral intake, with an associated rise in her serum albumin. Currently she is at home with her family, where she is symptom-free on medication. Because of her considerable symptomatic improvement she was keen to try further chemotherapy, and after discussion she was commenced on oral chlorambucil, which was felt to be the most appropriate option.

Case 3

This is a 53-year-old woman initially diagnosed with stage IIIc ovarian cancer in March 2001 for which she underwent initial debulking surgery, but was left with residual disease of up to 2 cm in the form of scattered peritoneal nodules. She underwent first-line combination chemotherapy (carboplatin, docetaxel, and gemcitabine on SCOTROC IIa trial) with radiological and Ca-125 response. However, within 3 months of finishing her chemotherapy, she relapsed with rapidly rising Ca-125 and CT appearance of recurrent peritoneal nodules up to 2.5 cm. It was felt that such a rapid, precipitous relapse after her initial chemotherapy suggested an aggressive highly resistant tumour, and options for second-line chemotherapy were discussed. The patient was referred for experimental treatment at a tertiary referral centre. She accepted entry into a phase II study of epothilone, with the knowledge that the treatment may not offer more likelihood of response than standard chemotherapy. Following two cycles of epothilone, the patient was shown to have progressive disease both on CT criteria and with rising Ca-125. She was offered various treatment options including further combination chemotherapy or newer chemotherapy drugs such as topotecan or liposomal doxorubicin (Caelyx), but eventually decided to receive the Van der Burg regimen of weekly cisplatin and oral etoposide. The patient tolerated this more intensive treatment surprisingly well—her main toxicities were haematological, requiring blood transfusions and eventually dose reduction. She also required aggressive magnesium supplementation for platinum-induced magnesium wasting nephropathy. Following the intensive phase of treatment, the patient had impressive improvements in her symptoms and palpable disease reduction. This was mirrored in a decline in Ca-125 from over 4000 to normal levels. Happily, the radiological appearances confirmed this excellent response with disappearance of much of the peritoneal disease. She remains symptom-free on maintenance oral etoposide, with a Ca-125 within the normal range and no radiological evidence of progression, 5 months on from her last cisplatin injection.

References

1 Ingelfinger, F. J. (1980). Arrogance. *N Engl J Med*, **303**(26), 1507–11.

2 Griffiths, C. T., Parker, L. M., Lee, S., and Finkler, N. J. (2002). The effect of residual mass size on response chemotherapy after surgical cytoreduction for advanced ovarian cancer: long-term results. *Int J Gynaecol Cancer*, **12**(4), 323–31.

3 Van der Burg, M. (2001). Advanced Ovarian Cancer. *Curr Treat Options Oncol*, **2**, 109–18.

4 The International Collaborative Ovarian Neoplasm (ICON) Group (2002). Paclitaxel plus carboplatin versus standard chemotherapy with single-agent carboplatin or

cyclophosphamide, doxorubicin, and cisplatin in women with ovarian cancer: the ICON 3 randomized trial. *Lancet*, **360**, 505–15.

5 McGuire, W. P., Hoskins, W. J., Brady, M. F. *et al.* (1996) Cyclophosphamide and cisplatin compared with paclitaxel and cisplatin in patients with stage III and IV ovarian cancer. *N Engl J Med*, **334**, 1–6.

6 Piccart, M. J., Bertelsen, K., James, K. *et al.* (2000). Randomized Intergroup trial of cisplatin-paclitaxel versus cisplatin-cyclophosphamide in women with advanced epithelial ovarian cancer: three-year results. *J Natl Cancer Inst*, **92**, 699–708.

7 Brenton, J. B., Earl, H. M., Caldas, C., Ahmed, A., Crawford, R., and Latimer, J. (2002). Expression profiling of advanced epithelial ovarian cancer to predict chemotherapy response. CTCR-OV01 (Cambridge Translational Cancer Research Study—OV01) *Cambridge LREC approved study protocol.*

8 Markman, M. (2001) Intraperitoneal chemotherapy in the management of malignant disease. *Expert Rev Anticancer Ther*, **1**,142–8.

9 Latorre, A., De Lena, M., Catino, A. *et al.* (2002). Epithelial ovarian cancer: second and third line chemotherapy (Review) *Int J Oncol*, **21**, 179–86.

10 Van der Burg, M., de Wit, R., van Putten, W. L. J. *et al.* (2002) Weekly cisplatin and daily oral etoposide is highly effective in platinum pretreated ovarian cancer. *Brit J Cancer*, **86**, 19–25.

11 Liu, B., Earl, H. M., Poole, C. J., Dunn, J., and Kerr, D. J. (1995). Etoposide protein binding in cancer patients. *Cancer Chemother Pharmacol*, **36**(6), 506–12.

12 Doyle, C., Crump, M., Pintilie, M., and Oza, A. M. (2001). Does palliative chemotherapy palliate? Evaluation of expectations, outcomes, and costs in women receiving chemotherapy for advanced ovarian cancer. *J Clin Oncol*, **19**, 1266–74.

13 Patnaik, A., Doyle, C., and Oza, A. M. (1998) Palliative chemotherapy in advanced ovarian cancer: balancing patient expectations, quality of life and cost. *Anticancer Drugs*, **9**, 869–78.

Chapter 3

Endometrial cancer: fundamentals and advanced disease

John J. Kavanagh

Epidemiology

Endometrial cancer is the most common gynaecological cancer in the United States and the second most common in the United Kingdom. It is predominantly a disease of the developed world. In 1999, 36 100 cases were diagnosed in the United States, and 6000 women died of their disease.[1] Altogether, 70% of endometrial cancers are found in post-menopausal women.

The major risk factors for endometrial cancer are the use of unopposed oestrogens or tamoxifen, nulliparity, obesity, hypertension, diabetes mellitus, and the presence of complex endometrial hyperplasia. For women taking tamoxifen, the degree of risk increases with increasing duration of use and has been calculated at 2.5 to 9 times higher than the normal population. Taking unopposed oestrogens results in a risk greater than 10 times that of the normal population. A woman who smokes or who uses the combined contraceptive pill reduces her chances of developing endometrial cancer. The risks of developing the other cancers associated with smoking are undiminished.

Presentation

The most common presenting symptom of endometrial cancer is vaginal bleeding and approximately 15% of post-menopausal women who have abnormal bleeding will prove to have endometrial carcinoma. The vast majority of women diagnosed with endometrial cancer will have noticed some sort of vaginal discharge.

If the disease is advanced, the patient may have both local and systemic symptoms. Locally advanced disease is associated with pelvic and back pain, symptoms of urinary tract obstructions secondary to obstructive nephropathy, and bleeding from the urinary tract or the rectum. Systemic symptoms may be associated with non-metastatic phenomena such as cachexia and fatigue and/or metastatic deposits. Occasionally patients present with ascites and other complaints consistent with peritoneal carcinomatosis[2] but other possible sites include the lungs, central nervous system, and bony skeleton.

Assessment

Post-menopausal women who complain of vaginal bleeding should have a histologic evaluation of the endometrial cavity. Out-patient sampling of the endometrial cavity with small catheters has largely replaced traditional dilatation and curettage. Both these techniques offer the same sensitivity for detecting hyperplasia or cancer. If out-patient sampling detects hyperplasia, or the examination is incomplete or unsatisfactory, then it is necessary to carry out dilatation and curettage (D&C) under a general anaesthetic.

The role of hysteroscopy remains controversial. The technique appears to offer superiority in detecting endometrial polyps and submucousal fibroids but it does not appear to be more sensitive in detecting malignancy. Hysteroscopy, however, may offer additional information about the extent of the disease.

The use of transvaginal ultrasound has also been advocated. It has a negative predictive value of nearly 100% if the thickness of the endometrium is considered normal. At a threshold of 5 mm it is extremely unlikely that the individual has significant pathology. However, this technique is not widely practiced.

Histology

Endometrioid adenocarcinoma represents over 75% of cases and can be graded from one to three with grade I being well differentiated, II—moderately differentiated, and III—poorly differentiated. The grading is based on the extent of loss of glandular formation. A difficulty arises when complex hyperplasia is present with atypia, also known as atypical hyperplasia. This entity appears to progress to carcinoma in 25% of cases. It may be confused with a grade I adenocarcinoma. Simple hyperplasia is a relatively benign disease with spontaneous regression in the order of 90%. However, one must be cautious, as samples are quite small with newer techniques and as many as 25% of atypical complex hyperplasia will have co-existing carcinoma.

Squamous metaplasia may be present with endometrial cancer and if it is extensive they are called adenoacanthomas. If the squamous component is malignant they are known as adenosquamous. Rare variants of the disease are papillary serous and clear cell, which represent about 15% of cases. These tend to be more aggressive and spread both systemically and locally.[3]

Uterine sarcomas are a rare entity classified as leiomyosarcomas, mixed mesodermal tumours, or endometrioid stromal sarcomas. The first two histological types often behave quite aggressively. The latter diagnosis is usually curable by surgery, but may recur locally.

Pretreatment evaluation

Endometrial cancers are currently staged surgically. A pre-operative chest radiograph is usually obtained. It is debatable whether any further radiographic imaging is necessary. In advanced cases, cystoscopy, sigmoido-scopy, and barium enema are reasonable procedures. In patients where one suspects that there is a possibility of metastatic disease, or if there is a poorly differentiated lesion, CT scanning of the abdomen and pelvis is a useful pre-operative investigation. The use of the MRI to determine myometrial invasion is being investigated and some consider it a practical tool for assessment. Mammograms are generally recommended pre-operatively. Anaemia, resulting from prolonged or heavy vaginal bleeding, is the most common abnormality on laboratory evaluation. The epithelial tumour marker Ca-125 is often produced by the malignancy, but its prognostic importance is uncertain.

Surgery

The surgical procedure combines staging with removal of the malignancy. The usual approach is exploratory laparotomy through a midline incision with total abdominal hysterectomy, and SOP (bilateral salpingo oophorectomy), pelvic washings, and inspection of the abdominal contents. It is essential to assess lymph node status for accurate staging. Lymphadenectomy, however, is not routinely performed. In patients who have a minimally invasive grade I cancer, the chances of finding a cancerous lymph node are so small that the morbidity is thought to exceed the benefit of the lymphadenectomy. A lymphadenectomy usually represents a sampling of the pelvic nodes and lower para-aortic nodes. The lymphadenectomy is tailored according to the risk of finding metastatic disease, body habitus of the patient, and underlying medical conditions that increase the risks of prolonged surgery.

The complication rate of surgery including lymphadenectomy is approxim-ately 5%, with the most common complication being post-operative thrombosis with a mortality of approximately 2%.

Staging

In 1988, The International Federation of Gynaecology and Obstetrics (FIGO) developed the surgical staging criteria utilizing the extent of:

(1) myometrial involvement;

(2) local extension; and

(3) involvement of lymph nodes.

The staging system is divided into stage I (uterine involvement); stage II (local extension involving the cervix, ovaries); stage III (regional lymph node disease, vaginal metastases, or positive peritoneal cytology); and stage IV (extensive regional involvement or distant metastasis). This is set out in Table 3.1. Staging is used to predict prognosis with stage I disease having a 75% 5-year survival, and stage IV approximately 10% survival at 5 years. It is clear that within each stage there are significant variations in survival, i.e. a stage I

Table 3.1 FIGO staging of endometrial cancer (Revised Surgical Staging 1988)

Stage	Grades	Description
Ia	I, II, III	Tumour limited to endometrium
Ib	I, II, III	Invasion to ≤50% myometrium
Ic	I, II, III	Invasion >50% myometrium
IIa	I, II, III	Endocervical glandular involvement only
IIb	I, II, III	Cervical stroma invasion
IIIa	I, II, III	Tumour invasion of serosa and/or adnexae, and/or positive peritoneal cytology
IIIb	I, II, III	Vaginal metastases
IIIc	I, II, III	Metastases to pelvic and/or para-aortic lymph nodes
IVa	I, II, III	Tumour invasion of bladder and/or bowel mucosa
IVb	I, II, III	Distant metastases, including intra-abdominal and/or inguinal lymph node

Unofficial designation: Stage II occult (cervical involvement noted by microscopic examination alone); for practical purposes, patients with stage I or stage II occult disease may be managed alike.
FIGO = International Federation of Gynecology and Obstetrics
Adapted from Beahrs O. H. *et al*: (1992) *Manual for staging of cancer*, p 162, Philadelphia: JB Lippincott.

patient with a grade I superficially invasive lesion has an almost 100% chance of survival: the majority of patients will have stage I disease (Table 3.2).[4, 5]

Treatment

Patients with stage I disease are treated by surgery unless they have medical conditions that contra-indicate the procedure: this should be exceptional now as there have been major improvements in medical support of such patients. Stage II patients usually undergo surgery if the disease is not too bulky in the cervical area: the procedure may be a radical hysterectomy or pre-operative cavitary radiation followed by hysterectomy and bilateral salpingo oophorectomy. Stage II endometrial cancers may be confused with adenocarcinoma of the cervix. Stage III and IV diseases are unusual and the approach must be tailored to the individual patient. The presence of serosal involvement usually requires post-operative radiotherapy. Surgical extirpation and radiation are used if vaginal metastases are present. Every patient with stage IV disease must be assessed and treated individually, depending on the severity of their pain, the degree of bleeding, and the extent of metastatic disease. Any of the following techniques may be used alone or in combination: surgical bulk reduction, palliative radiation to control pelvic symptoms, and systemic chemotherapy.

Radiotherapy[6, 7]

Patients who have stage I high-grade disease and/or deep invasion of myometrium are treated with post-operative radiotherapy to reduce the chances of recurrence within the vaginal vault. It does not improve survival but does reduce the incidence of local and regional recurrence. Radiotherapy

Table 3.2 Distribution of patients by stage at presentation and respective survival rates

Stage	Percent at diagnosis	% Survival at 5 yr
I	74.8	76.3
II	11.4	59.2
III	10.7	29.4
IV	2.9	10.3
Unstaged	0.2	51.8
Overall	100.0	66.9

Adapted from Hacker NF: Uterine cancer, in Berek JS, Hacker NF (eds): Practical Gynecologic Oncology, 2nd ed. pp 285–326. Baltimore, Williams & Wilkins, 1994.

is also given to individuals who have involvement of pelvic or lower para-aortic lymph nodes, poor prognosis histologies, and involvement of the ovaries. Radiotherapy to the pelvis is usually given as a combination of external beam and brachytherapy treatment applied locally to the vaginal vault. Care will be taken to limit the radiation dose to the bladder and bowel as much as possible. The complications of pelvic radiotherapy include vaginal stenosis, radiation cystitis, and proctitis. Small bowel obstruction and rectosigmoid stricture are possible delayed complications.

Hormonal therapy

There is no evidence that adjuvant hormonal therapy is of any benefit in endometrial cancer. There is no dose–response relationship, nor is there a particular method of administration which is superior.

Patients who are most likely to respond to progestational compounds include thosewith:

- well differentiated tumours;
- treatment free intervals of more than one year;
- pulmonary metastases; and
- slowly growing tumours.

Patients with higher-grade tumours have a less than 10% response rate. Tamoxifen and gonadotropin agonists have also produced a partial response in some patients.

Chemotherapy[8]

Chemotherapy is an option for patients considered unsuitable for hormonal therapy. Its use is strictly for palliation. The drugs utilized are shown in Table 3.3. Most physicians advise either single-agent carboplatin or a combination of a platin with doxorubicin or paclitaxel. Response rates are greater with distant disease, particularly pulmonary metastasis. The response rates are approximately 20–50%, with a median duration of response of 4–8 months. Patients who start chemotherapy have a median survival of less than 12 months.

Palliative care issues

Patients with refractory endometrial cancer are likely to have two particular palliative care problems (Table 3.4). The first issue is local recurrence that may cause bleeding, pain, lympho-oedema secondary to tumour obstruction, and thrombosis. Fortunately this tends to be less common than it once was, as

Table 3.3 Active chemotherapy agents

Drug	Response (%)
Doxorubicin	19–38
Cisplatin	4–42
Carboplatin	32
Cyclophosphamide	0–20
Ifosfamide	13
Fluorouracil	24
Hexamethylmelamine	9–30
Paclitaxel*	35

Adapted from Thigpen JT: Chemotherapy of cancers of the female genital tract, in Perry MC (ed): The Chemotherapy Source Book, Ist ed. pp 1039–1067. Baltimore, Williams & Wilkins, 1992, and Thigpen J et al: Cancer 60:2104–2116, 1987.

* Ball HG: Personal communications, Fifth Biennial Meeting of the International Gynecologic Cancer Society, September, 1995.

Table 3.4 Palliative care issues

Local recurrences	
Pelvic bleeding	– Fatigue
Fistulae	– Local skin mucosal irritation
	– Social embarrassment and isolation
Mass effect	– Pelvic pain
	– Bladder/bowel compression
Distant recurrence	
Lymph nodes	– Back pain
	– Neck pain
Carcinomatosis	– Abdominal swelling
	– Poor appetite
	– Nausea/vomiting
Lung/pelvic	– Cough
	– Shortness of breath
Brain (late)	– Neurologic dysfunction
Skeleton	– Bony Pain
	– Fractures

patients tend to present earlier in the course of their disease and because of improvements in primary therapy. The second and most common group of palliative care problems is related to distant disease. The most common sites of metastases requiring palliative care intervention are bone, brain, and retroperitoneal lymph nodes. Occasionally patients will present with ascites and carcinomatosis mimicking the problems of ovarian cancer. Rapidly growing pulmonary metastases will cause cough and shortness of breath.

Conclusion

Cancer of the uterus is most commonly found in post-menopausal women and presents as vaginal bleeding, accompanied by vaginal discharge. Women at particular risk are those who have unopposed oestrogen therapy, obesity, nulliparity, and diabetes. The diagnosis is usually obtained by small catheter aspiration of the endometrial cavity. If necessary, a formal dilatation and curettage should be performed. Once diagnosed, the pre-operative work-up usually involves a chest X-ray and mammogram. CT scans of the abdomen and pelvis are used in patients who have a higher grade lesion or suspicion of distant metastasis including lymph nodes. The surgery is a combination of a staging procedure and extirpation of the gynaecologic organs. Following surgery, post-operative radiotherapy is given to those who are considered at risk for local recurrence, i.e. higher grade lesions or those involving significant in parts of the myometrium. The use of hormonal therapy and chemotherapy is reserved for those who develop metastatic disease or regional recurrences not amenable to surgery or further radiotherapy. The most common sites of metastatic disease are the lungs, brain, and bones: occasionally patients develop painful retroperitoneal lymphadenopathy.

References

1   Horowitz, I. R. (2001). *Obstetrics and gynaecology clinics of North America: gynaecologic oncology for the generalist,* 28(4). Philadelphia: W.B. Saunders Company.

2   Shafi, M. I., Luesley, D. M., and Jordan, J. A. (2001). *Handbook of gynaecological oncology.* London: Churchill Livingstone.

3   Dunton, C., Balsara, G., McFarland, M. *et al.* (1991). Uterine papillary serous carcinoma: a review. *Obstet Gynaecol Surv,* **46**, 97–102.

4   Morrow, C. P., Bundy, B. N., Kurman, R. J. *et al.* (1991). Relationship between surgical-pathological risk factors and outcome in clinical stage I and II carcinoma of the endometrium: a gynaecologic oncology group study. *Gynaecol Oncol,* **40**, 55–65.

5   Yazigi, R., Piver, M. S., and Blumenson, I. (1983). Malignant peritoneal cytology as a prognostic indicator in stage I endometrial cancer. *Obstet Gynaecol,* **62**, 359–362.

6   Ackerman, I., Malone, S., Thomas, G. *et al.* (1996). Endometrial carcinoma: relative effectiveness of adjuvant irradiation vs. therapy reserved for relapse. *Gynaecol Oncl,* **60**, 177–183.

7   Kucera, H., Vavra, N., and Weghaupt, K. (1990). Benefits of external irradiation in pathologic stage I endometrial carcinoma: a prospective clinical trial of 605 patients who received postoperative vaginal irradiation and additional pelvic irradiation in the presence of unfavorable prognostic factors. *Gynaecol Oncol*, **38**, 99–104.

8   Zanotti, K. M., Belinson, J. L., Kennedy, A. W. *et al.* (1999). The use of paclitaxel and platinum-based chemotherapy in uterine papillary serous carcinoma. *Gynaecol Oncol*, **74**, 272–277.

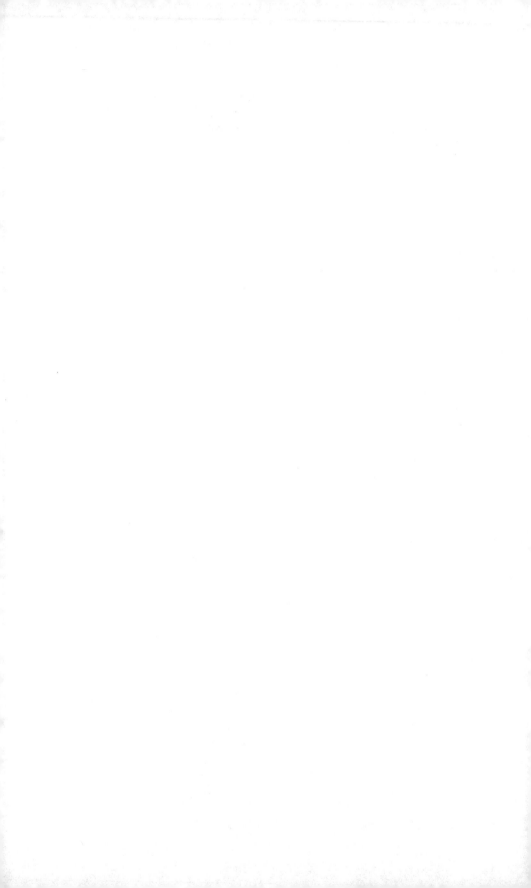

Chapter 4

Pelvic pain syndromes and their management in advanced gynaecological malignancy

Sebastiano Mercadante

Introduction

Gynaecological malignancies constitute approximately 20% of visceral cancers in women. Locally advanced cancers in the pelvis produce progressive pelvic and perineal pain, as well as other complications, including ureteric obstruction with uraemia, and lymphatic and venous obstruction. Invasion of the tumour into the rectum or bladder can lead to erosion with bleeding, sloughing of tumour into the urine or bowel, and bladder or bowel outlet obstruction.

Ovarian cancer is associated with recurrent episodes of bowel obstruction, para-neoplastic syndromes including peripheral neuropathies, and disturbances of the CNS, all of which can cause severe pain.

Oncological treatments may cause significant anatomical and functional damage, and even patients with advanced disease may receive one or more of the chemotherapeutic regimens currently in use. Serious local problems can develop as a result of neurotoxic chemotherapy, external beam radiation, radiation implants, hysterectomy, vulvectomy, vaginectomy, pelvic exenteration, and other treatments. Pain is the most frequently reported symptom complicating therapy.

This chapter focuses on the pathophysiology and pharmacological treatment of pelvic pain in gynaecological malignancy—the *basic* principles of palliative care are not discussed. The management of pain accompanying bowel obstruction is discussed in Chapter 7.

It should always be remembered that pain is a somato-psychic experience and the social, psychological, and spiritual aspects of pain need the same attention as the medical, if pain is to be managed effectively. Pain management cannot be achieved without an understanding of the pathophysiology of pelvic pain syndromes and this needs to be integrated with general palliative care management to achieve the best possible pain control.

Table 4.1 Causes of pain in patients with gynaecological malignancies—in order of incidence

1. Direct nerve damage caused by tumour infiltration or inflammatory changes in the pelvis
2. Compression of adjacent structures by enlarging tumour masses
3. Neuropathies due to treatment of the cancer (post-surgical, post-radiotherapy, or neurotoxic chemotherapy)
4. Malignant invasion of sacral bone or distant metastases
5. Peri-tumoural oedema, infection, or necrosis surrounding adjacent structures
6. Obstruction of hollow viscus by tumour
7. Malignant invasion of the rich muscular structure of the pelvis
8. Vascular occlusion
9. Manifestations of paraneoplastic syndromes

There are many causes of pain in patients with gynaecological malignancy—for example:

♦ lumbar pain due to iliopsoas muscle involvement;

♦ nerve trunk pain, often radiating to lower limbs due to the involvement of lumbosacral plexus;

♦ tumour involvement in the pre-sacral area;

♦ radiculopathy related to retroperitoneal spread.

A full list is set out in Table 4.1.

Anatomy

The pelvis is an inverted truncated cone continuous with the abdominal cavity. It contains viscera, muscles, ligaments and joints, vessels and nodes, nerves, and the skeleton of the pelvis. It is bordered by the pubic crest and the obturator muscle anterolaterally, sacrum, coccyx, and piriform muscle posterosuperiorly, and inferiorly by the muscles of perineal floor. The viscera within the pelvis are supplied by sympathetic and parasympathetic nerves that contain both afferent and efferent fibres. The superior hypogastric plexus is situated in front of the bifurcation of the abdominal aorta. At its lower border, the plexus divides into the right and left hypogastric plexus. It gives off branches to the ureteral and testicular or ovarian plexuses, the body of uterus and the cervix, and supplies the transverse colon, splenic flexure, and descending colon. The inferior hypogastric plexus supplies pelvic organs including the rectum, urinary bladder, prostate, uterus, and vagina. The pudendal nerve, branches of ilioinguinal, genitofemoral, and anococcygeal nerves innervate the perineum.[1]

Mechanisms of pain

Different pathophysiological mechanisms underlie different clinical pain syndromes. The pain syndromes associated with gynaecological malignancy are related to the characteristics and progression of the underlying disease including the preferential sites of metastases, which vary with each primary site. In order to develop rational, clinical treatment strategies for each pain that a patient suffers, it is important to have an understanding of the neurophysiological changes that cause them.

Cancer pain classification

Pain related to malignant disease can be classified as nociceptive (somatic and visceral) and neuropathic.

Somatic and visceral pains involve *direct* activation of nociceptors, and often complicate infiltration of tissue by tumour or tissue damage as a consequence of oncological treatments.

Neuropathic pain may be a complication of injury to the peripheral or central nervous system and is often poorly tolerated and difficult to control.

Temporal patterns of pain

The following terms describe different patterns of pain. Whatever the cause of the pain the clinician needs a good understanding of its timing in order to treat it effectively.

Breakthrough pain

This term refers to intermittent exacerbations of pain that can occur spontaneously or in relation to specific activity, especially at the end of the dosing interval of the regularly scheduled analgesic.

Incident pain

This is a sort of breakthrough pain. Some pains may be only moderately severe or absent whilst the patient is at rest but are exacerbated by different movements or positions, such as standing, walking, sitting, turning, deep breathing, coughing or with pressure on the area of involvement—this is called incident pain.

Incident pain is a very difficult to manage successfully as although the exacerbation associated with movement can be very short–lived it is often very severe and incapacitating for the patient. For example, a bed-bound patient with a fractured neck of femur may develop bedsores in their anxiety to keep absolutely still because of severe short-lived pain provoked by movement.

Incident pain is not always preventable, even if predictable. It is the best known type of breakthrough pain and is commonly caused by bone metastases or is found in association with neuropathic pain (see below).

Nociceptive pain

No specific histological structure acts as a nociceptive receptor. A-delta and C-fibres have been clearly identified as having high-threshold transducers, which become involved as the intensity of the injuring stimulus increases. A repeated and intense stimulus induces the release of several inflammatory mediators, which may:

♦ reduce the threshold for activation;

♦ increase the response to a given stimulus; or

♦ induce the appearance of spontaneous activity.

Various chemicals are released into damaged tissue cells. Substance P is able to induce the production of nitrous oxide, a vasodilatator, and the degranulation of mast cells with a further vasodilatation and subsequent extravasation and release of bradykinin. The enhanced release of substance P and other neurokinins may be the reason that the NMDA receptor for the excitatory amino acids becomes more easily activated. These transmitters together activate spinal cord neurones. The activation of NMDA receptors will result in an amplification of the response underlying central hyperalgesia. The repetition of a constant intensity C-fibre stimulus induces the phenomenon of "wind-up", that is a switch from a low-level of pain-related activity to a high level without any change in the inputs arriving in the peripheral nerves. It has been suggested that nitric oxide (NO) feeds back to increase the release of C-fibre transmitters, further enhancing pain transmission.[2]

Somatic pain

Somatic pain is caused by stimulation of nociceptors by direct extension of the tumour through fascial planes and their lymphatic supplies. Nociceptors are found in the integument and supporting structures, i.e. striated muscles, joints, bones (including periosteum), and nerve trunks. Pain is the result of somatosensory input generated by sensory signals from these tissues. Somatic pain is usually well localized and constant. Deep somatic pain is associated with cutaneous hyperalgesia, tenderness, reflex muscle spasm, and sympathetic hyperactivity.

Bone pain Bone metastases are a major problem in advanced cancer and frequently give rise to complications that can have a devastating impact on the woman's quality of life. Complications include difficulty walking, even complete immobility, neurological deficits, and pathological fractures.

Table 4.2 Cancer pain syndromes associated with direct tumour involvement of vertebral bodies in gynaecological malignancy

Vertebral body syndrome	Symptoms and signs
T12-L1 syndrome NB: imaging of pelvic bones alone will miss cause of pain, need soft tissue too.	Dull aching, mid-back pain exacerbated by lying or sitting, relieved by standing. Pain can radiate in girdle-like band anteriorly or to both paraspinal and lumbrosacral area. May be referred to sacroiliac joint and superior iliac crest.
Sacral syndrome	Destruction of sacrum leads to severe, aching, focal pain in low back or coccygeal area, radiating to buttocks, perineum or posterior thighs. Insidious onset. Exacerbated by lying, sitting, relieved by walking. Increasing pain with perianal sensory loss. Bowel, bladder dysfunction may develop. Lateral extension may cause incident pain in hip. Local invasion of sacral plexus may occur.

(Adapted from Stannard, C. F. and Booth, S. (1998). *A pocket book of pain*, 1st edn. Churchill Livingstone.

Incident pain (see above), which is frequently associated with bone metastases, is usually difficult to control with drug therapy alone. It is important to warn patients that complete control of pain is difficult when there is a component of incident pain.[3]

Direct tumour involvement of the pelvic bony skeleton is also possible in advanced gyanecological malignancy: various syndromes have been described (Table 4.2).

Mechanisms of bone pain The resorption of bone as a result of increased osteoclastic activation decreases bone density and disrupts skeletal architecture, either focally or throughout the skeleton. Periosteum is usually very pain-sensitive, as the density of myelinated and unmyelinated afferent fibres is high. Microfractures may occur in bony trabeculae at the site of metastases resulting in bone distortion.

Pain occurs because of one or more of the following:

♦ the stretching of periosteum by tumour expansion;

♦ mechanical stress of the weakened bone;

♦ nerve entrapment by the tumour; or

♦ direct destruction of the bone with consequent collapse

Bone pain typically develops insidiously over a period of weeks or months, becoming progressively more severe. The pain is characteristically described as dull, constant, and of gradually increasing intensity. Moreover, pain from bone metastases can produce a variety of symptoms.[4]

Bone metastases and breakthrough pain Internal fixation and radiotherapy are central to the management of bone metastases but the former may not be possible because the patient is too ill and there may be a delay in providing the latter. Patients with pain from bone metastases on weight-bearing or movement, may require a dose of opioid that causes excessive adverse effects for the patient at rest, as movement-related pain is likely to be repetitive and in some cases unpredictable.

A specialist pain/palliative care opinion is usually needed as spinal analgesia or a nerve block may be required.

Visceral pain

Pelvic viscera have complex innervation from the peripheral nervous system. Visceral nociceptors have a wide range of responses, and may be activated in the presence of inflammation or tissue injury. Therefore, visceral afferents are considered polymodal, giving excitatory response to different stimuli, including inflammation, stretching, and distension.[5]

Neurones that transmit visceral sensory information to the spinal cord have cell bodies in the dorsal root ganglia. These primary afferents travel through the para-vertebral ganglia, through the pre-vertebral ganglia from the sensory endings in the viscera themselves. Afferent fibres travel in conjunction with motor fibres of parasympathetic and sympathetic nervous system. Most visceral afferents have relatively slow conduction velocities.

Visceral pain tends to be diffuse because of the absence of a separate visceral sensory pathway and the low proportion of visceral afferent nerve fibres compared with those of somatic origin. Thus, the neurological mechanisms responsible for visceral pain differ from those involved in somatic pain. Most solid viscera are not sensitive to pain, and some stimuli, such as cutting, may be less painful than expected. Pain is diffuse, poorly localized and can be referred to other anatomic locations—'referred pain'—and is often associated with motor and autonomic reflexes. One common example is shoulder pain due to diaphragmatic irritation from large subdiaphragmatic masses in ovarian cancer. Gross abdominal distension, from ascites, may also induce shoulder pain and hiccough.

Better localization of painful stimuli occur when the disease involves a somatically innervated structure such as the parietal peritoneum.

Other painful stimuli Mechanical stimuli, such as torsion or traction of mesenteries, distension of hollow organs, stretch of serosal and mucosal surfaces, and compression of some organs is painful. These conditions are frequently observed in patients with advanced pelvic malignancies.

Renal colic Ureteric obstruction in the pelvis is common in advanced cervical cancer and the distension of the ureter and renal pelvis causes renal colic. Pain is also related to pressure in the urinary bladder.

Movement of the bladder or bowel may also induce colicky breakthrough pain in patients whose analgesic regimen is generally satisfactory.

Ischaemic pain Ischaemic pain occurs particularly in tissues involved in metastatic disease or those recently damaged by surgery. Ischaemia may act as a modulator of mechanoreceptive visceral inputs. The variability of response to ischaemia may be due to any pre-existing pathology or to cancer-related mechanical distortion of the pelvic organ secondary to local changes.

These models of visceral pain help to explain a disappointing result from some neurolytic blocks given for pelvic cancer pain or a poor response to analgesic drugs. Failure or partial success of a hypogastric plexus block may be attributed to the fact the tumour has metastasized beyond the nerves that conduct pain via the plexus and the component nerves that form it.

Neuropathic pain

Neuropathic pain is defined as pain resulting from damage to the peripheral or central nervous systems. It most commonly occurs as a consequence of tumour compression or infiltration of nerves contained in the pelvis, or nervous structures close to the sacrum.

Many patients with advanced gynaecological malignancy develop neuropathic pain: due to nerve damage or sensory loss that is described as numbness, burning, crawling sensation, and tightness.

Neuropathic pain is associated with some characteristic symptoms such as:

allodynia—pain which follows a normally innocuous stimulus such as light touch;

hyperalgesia—pain of abnormal severity following a noxious stimulus;

hyperpathia—increased pain in an area of increased sensory threshold.

Neuropathic pain has a variable onset, as it can be continuous, spontaneous, or paroxysmal.

It has been suggested that hyperalgesia reflects a sensitization of receptors, while allodynia is a central phenomenon mediated by large myelinated fibres. Pain may be either superficial or deep. Referred and abnormal pain radiation, such as the presence of abnormal sensations and pain over large areas of skin, are typically observed in myelopathies. The degree of radiation and referral is likely a reflection of a progressive recruiting of wide range neurones in deeper layers of the dorsal horn. Moreover, an increased activity is seen in sympathetic efferents following sensitization of C-nociceptors with spontaneous discharges in C-fibres and maintained in part by alpha-1 receptors.

Some common neuropathic pain syndromes are illustrated in Table 4.3.

Aetiology of neuropathic pain in gynaecological malignancy

Direct nerve infiltration The abundant nerve supply to the pelvis is vulnerable to direct malignant infiltration which can result in, for example, lumbosacral plexopathies from the invasion of perineal nerves. This causes poorly localized dull aching pain in the thighs (for example) and may be accompanied by symptomatic sensory loss, causalgia, and deafferentation syndromes (see Table 4.3).

Direct pressure on nerves by metastatic disease Metastatic disease may cause lumbrosacral plexopathies, spinal cord or cauda equina syndromes.

Table 4.3 Cancer pain syndromes in advanced gynaecological malignancy caused by direct nerve infiltration

Nerve(s) infiltrated by tumour	Symptoms and signs
Lumbrosacral plexopathy Associated with local extension of advanced gynaecological malignancy including sarcomas plus other primary sites e.g. NHL Lumbar plexus: L1–4: (anterior primary rami) lies on paravertebral psoas muscle.	Pain earliest symptom, dull, aching, constant. Upper plexopathy (30% pts) c/o pain in back, lower abdomen, flank, iliac crest, anterolateral thigh. Sensory symptoms/signs in L1–4 distribution. May also have pain on flexion of ipsilateral hip ('malignant psoas syndrome.')
Sacral plexus = L4–5 trunk & S1–3 (anterior primary rami)	Lower plexopathy most common >50% patients. Usually pelvic tumours. Pain in buttocks, perineum, posterolateral part of the leg. May have sensory changes and weakness in L5-S1 distribution. Bladder and bowel dysfunction and leg oedema may be present.
Sacral plexopathy Occurs frequently in patients with advanced gynaecological malignancy also common in colonic and genito-urinary malignancy. NB CT/MRI scanning necessary to assess lumbrosacral plexopathy	Dull, aching midline pain. Local extension of a sacral/presacral mass. Sensory loss beginning in presacral area. Sensory findings commonly unilateral at first then progressing to bilateral sacral sensory loss and autonomic dysfunction. Numbness over dorsal medial foot and sole, weakness of ankle dorsiflexion and inversion. Bladder and bowel dysfunction possible. Patient may be unable to lie or sit down because of pain.

Adapted from Stannard, C. F. and Booth, S. *A pocketbook of pain*, 1st edn, (1998) pp 231. Churchill Livingstone.

Viral infections All patients with advanced cancer are immunocompromised by the effects of the underlying disease. This may be compounded by drug therapy such as corticosteroids.

Rectal neuralgia from herpes zoster is the cause of a well-recognized syndrome, proctalgia fugax.

Adverse effects of drugs used in chemotherapy Mono- and polyneuropathies, may be induced by vincristine, paclitaxel, and cisplatin therapy. Pain is characterized by paraesthesia distally and neurological changes such as arreflexia and sensory changes may be found on examination. Patients may walk with a wide-based gait because of loss of proprioception—the pain can be very severe and resistant to standard therapies for neuropathic pain. The pain frequently resolves, at least partially, over months, sometimes years.

Radiation-induced nerve damage Radiation can produce many of the same clinical pain syndromes as the disease itself but these occur months or years after the original treatment and they have become much more unusual as it has become possible to give lower total doses using longer courses of smaller fractions with much more precision.

Neuropathic cancer pain is varied in presentation, irreversible, and difficult to treat. Once established, neuropathic pain (with accompanying spinal hyper-excitability) is independent of the afferent input: this is why it is so difficult to control.

The multiple mechanisms underlying the pathophysiology of neuropathic pain may explain the differential sensitivity to opioids, as different nerve injuries and the dynamic course of the illness initiate varying degrees of neuronal plasticity and influence the responsiveness to opioids.[6]

Treatment

The current treatment of nociceptive pain is based on the WHO analgesic ladder, which sets out a graduated approach to the use of analgesic drugs: it is a framework of principles rather than a rigid protocol (see Fig. 4.1).

Step 1: Pharmacological studies have demonstrated that a broad spectrum of analgesics is effective in cancer pain. NSAIDs are the drugs commonly used as first step of the analgesic ladder and their usefulness for both somatic and visceral pain has been demonstrated. They are also effective in combination with opioids, regardless of the pain mechanism involved. NSAIDs have been shown to have useful opioid-sparing effects in long-term studies and to maintain this for prolonged periods of time.[7]

Steps 2 and 3 of the analgesic ladder: When cancer patients experience severe pain, opioids are the mainstay of therapy.[8] There are many ways of delivering

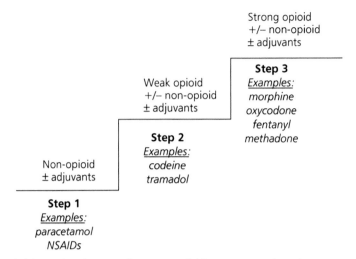

Opioids are agonists at endogenous opioid receptors, such as the mu receptor, producing 'morphine-like' activity.

Adjuvants are additional drugs that can be used as part of pain management, such as secondary analgesics (eg. gabapentin for neuropathic pain) and drugs to control analgestic adverse effects.

Fig. 4.1 WHO three-step analgesic ladder.

opioids in the management of cancer pain. In some clinical situations, there are clear indications for using one preparation or delivery system over another; for example:

- the potential or actual complications associated with that system;
- the efficacy of that system to deliver acceptable analgesia;
- the ability of the patient to use a specific type of delivery system;
- the complications associated with that system;
- the ease of use for the patient and her family; and
- cost is another important consideration both for those patients who purchase their own medication and for health care providers which, across the world, are under pressure to contain costs.

Oral route

The oral route is the one most commonly used. It has several advantages—it is the safest, the least invasive, the least expensive, and the easiest route for opioid administration for most patients with cancer pain. *In all patients who can take oral medication, this route should be considered first.* The main problem with the oral route is the first-pass biotransformation of opioids in the liver. All opioids given orally are absorbed via the gastric and duodenal mucosa and then transported to the liver via the portal venous system. In the liver, the drugs undergo 'first-pass metabolism' before entering the systemic circulation. As there is huge inter-individual variation in the degree of first-pass metabolism, conversion between oral and parenteral routes can only be approximate. After making a change the patient requires careful monitoring for signs of inadequate analgesia or a relative overdose of opioid.

First-pass metabolism has a major impact on the systemic plasma concentrations of drugs. For example, the dose of morphine given orally to a patient with cancer pain must be two to three times the intravenous or subcutaneous dose. This is true of other opioids.

Oxycodone is roughly equipotent to morphine if given parenterally, but appears to be approximately twice as potent as morphine when given orally because of less first-pass metabolism.

Modified-release preparations

Morphine is the most commonly used medication in the world to treat moderate to severe cancer pain. As it has a short duration of effect when used in an 'immediate release' form, several preparations have become available to provide longer lasting analgesia. Bioavailability of these modified-release preparations is the same as that of immediate-release preparations, but time to peak plasma drug concentrations is longer, and peak plasma concentration is decreased. Recommendations for most of these preparations state that they should be administered every 12 h. Clinicians occasionally use an 8-h schedule, if necessary, to provide adequate analgesia, but this is not standard practice. There are other preparations, such as a morphine pellet coated with a polymer, which can be administered once every 24 h.

Specific issues with breakthrough pain

If additional opioid analgesia is needed for 'breakthrough' pain, doses of a fast-onset, short-acting opioid preparation should be available to the patient. However, most immediate-release oral opioid preparations take approximately 30 min to the onset of analgesic action when taken on an empty stomach, and faster routes may be required, such as the subcutaneous or transmucosal routes (see below).

The rescue dose

A rescue dose of opioid can provide a means of treating breakthrough pain in patients already stabilized on a baseline opioid regimen. The use of an opioid, with short half-life, such as immediate-release morphine or hydromorphone, is suggested. The size of the most effective dose remain unknown, although clinicians suggest a dose roughly equivalent to 5–10% of the total opioid dose administered as needed every 2–3 h. (*Editor's note*: one-sixth of total 24-h dose is standard in UK at present.) However, the onset of action of an oral dose may be too slow (more than 30 min) and better results may be obtained with a parenteral rescue dose. Although the intravenous route is the fastest, subcutaneous administration is associated with an acceptable onset of effect and should be considered equivalent in terms of efficacy. PCA may be an option for both routes.

Fentanyl lozenges

Oral transmucosal dosing is a recent non-invasive approach to the rapid onset of analgesia. Highly lipophylic agents may pass rapidly through the oral mucosa avoiding the first-pass metabolism achieving active plasma concentrations within minutes. Fentanyl, incorporated in a hard matrix on a handle, is rapidly absorbed. It has been shown to have an onset of pain relief similar to intravenous morphine that is within 10–15 min. When the fentanyl matrix dissolves, approximately 25% of the total fentanyl concentration crosses the buccal mucosa and enters the bloodstream. The remaining amount is swallowed and about one-third of this part is absorbed, thus achieving a total bioavailability of 50%. Different controlled studies have shown the effectiveness of oral transmucosal fentanyl for treating episodes of breakthrough pain.

> It is important to stress that the effective transmucosal dose is not correlated with the basal analgesic regimen of transdermal fentanyl, underlining the need to individualize the dose.[9]

Switching opioid

Different opioids have different effects on the subsets of opioid receptors in the central nervous system and 'cross tolerance' between opioids is incomplete. This can be exploited when the adverse effects of one particular opioid are making it unacceptable to an individual as an analgesic and cannot be controlled. In these circumstances a change from one opioid to another is sometimes a useful option. Oxycodone, methadone, and hydromorphone are possible alternatives to oral morphine.

Methadone

Methadone in particular, has interesting extra-opioid properties, such as inhibition of NMDA receptors, which are useful in giving additional analgesia and a low rate of tolerance.

The degree of cross-tolerance may change as the dose of opioid is increased and care must be taken in applying an equi-analgesic dose formula to patients on high doses of any opioid, but this is particularly important when switching them to methadone.[10] Moreover, methadone's potency may be much greater than expected when a switch is made from another opioid because tolerance is reversed, probably due to its anti-NMDA effect. *Methadone should only be used by specialists or on specialist advice.*

> Strict surveillance is necessary when converting patients taking high doses of one opioid to another drug in the same class.

Adverse effects

Patients will develop tolerance to most of the undesirable side-effects of opioids (such as nausea/vomiting or sedation) over a period of several days. Tolerance rarely develops to constipation but there is great inter-individual variation in the severity of this symptom and the amount of treatment it requires.

If patients continue to have unacceptable adverse effects in spite of active management and appropriate use of opioids, it may be necessary to use another opioid of equivalent efficacy.

Parenteral route

The oral route is not suitable for every patient. Possible reasons include:

- oesophageal motility problems (e.g. head and neck cancer, oesophageal cancer);
- gastro-intestinal obstruction (bowel obstruction from ovarian cancer);
- uncontrollable nausea and vomiting (e.g. bowel obstruction);
- swallowing difficulties because of the site of their cancer (e.g. head and neck cancer);
- co-existing non-malignant conditions such as neurological impairment;
- being unconscious, comatose or very drowsy—most dying patients who have been on regular analgesics will require them parenterally to give good symptom control when they can no longer take drugs by mouth.

In these situations alternative routes such as subcutaneous, intravenous and transdermal should be considered.[8]

Subcutaneous route

This simple method of parenteral administration is now commonly used in palliative care and has largely replaced other alternative routes to oral administration where syringe drivers are available. It involves inserting a small plastic cannula under the skin of the chest, abdomen, upper arms, or thighs and attaching the tubing to an infusion pump.

Drugs may be administered as a bolus or continuous infusion. A subcutaneous opioid takes about 20 min to start having an effect reaching a peak within 40 min: the duration of action depends on the half-life of the drug.

The limiting factor for continuous subcutaneous infusion is the volume of fluid that can be injected per hour and concentrated solutions of drugs are helpful.

Most drugs used by intravenous route can also be used by the subcutaneous route, although pain and irritation are possible with methadone.

Advantages of the subcutaneous route include:

◆ no need for intravascular access;
◆ changing sites of infusion can be easily accomplished;
◆ dangerous infection and the other complications of the intravenous route can be avoided.

Disadvantages include:

◆ need for subcutaneous pump, which is relatively costly and needs correct maintenance;
◆ may need two pumps to deliver drugs which would be incompatible in the same syringe.

The subcutaneous syringe driver has been a great advance in palliative care in the last 30 years—before its widespread use many dying patients had to be given four hourly injections to maintain their comfort in their last days or hours.

Intravenous route

This is indicated for those patients:

◆ whose pain cannot be controlled by a less invasive route;
◆ who already have central venous access;
◆ who need parenteral medication but have very low platelet counts.

It is mostly used in haematology patients and will not often be used for patients with advanced gynaecological malignancy.

Advantages include:

◆ rapid onset of action allowing for an almost immediate effect in emergency conditions;
◆ no first-pass metabolism therefore more predictable dosing requirements;
◆ consistent delivery—poor peripheral perfusion can reduce the amount of drug absorbed when subcutaneous/intramuscular routes are used.

Disadvantages include:

◆ it is complex to manage and requires a higher level of training in professional staff, which makes it less easy, but not impossible, to use in home care;

- bolus doses of opioids (or benzodiazepines) can cause respiratory depression;
- the equipment is needed to deliver intravenous (IV) drugs is more expensive and elaborate;
- the speed of administration must be particularly carefully controlled;
- infection of central or peripheral venous lines can be very uncomfortable and may cause life-threatening infections—this is a particular risk for the immunosuppressed.

A number of opioids are available in intravenous solution in most countries, including morphine, hydromorphone, fentanyl, alfentanil, sufentanil, and methadone.

Fentanyl and sufentanil

Fentanyl is approximately 80–100 times more potent than morphine, and sufentanil is approximately 1000 times more potent.

Advantages include:

- lower incidence of constipation, nausea, vomiting and sedation than morphine;
- low incidence of histamine release;
- low incidence of other adverse drug reactions;
- no active metabolites;
- useful in renal impairment because of absence of active metabolites and mostly excreted from GI tract

Disadvantages include:

- high cost compared to morphine;
- smaller range of different preparations available;
- fentanyl is not suitable for routine IV administration, as it is a potent respiratory depressant

Patient-controlled analgesia (PCA)

Intravenous or subcutaneous opioid infusions can be given as continuous infusions or by a patient-controlled analgesia (PCA) device, which provides a continuous infusion plus on-demand boluses. The PCA device should be set initially to deliver a continuous infusion with the bolus dose at 25% of the hourly dose and with a lock-out interval of 2 h. The bolus dose should be adjusted to provide supplementary analgesia, to counter or minimize breakthrough pain. 'Lock-out' intervals should be modified on the basis of clinical need.

Contra-indications to using a PCA:

+ cognitive impairment;
+ patients dislike of the technical aspects of PCA;
+ patients who exhibit drug-seeking behaviour.

PCA has other drawbacks—it is invasive and it is associated with all the other complications inherent in the long-term use of subcutaneous needles or intravenous lines. The pump itself may limit patient mobility and the team caring for the patient requires a higher level of technical expertise.

The oral—parenteral ratio for morphine is 2:1 or 3:1.[8]

Transdermal route

This is another non-invasive way of maintaining a continuous plasma concentration of opioid.

Fentanyl

A fentanyl patch consist of a reservoir of fentanyl (sufficient for about three days) in combination with alcohol. The patch releases fentanyl at a constant rate until the reservoir is depleted. Upon initial application of the patch, a subcutaneous 'depot' is formed as fentanyl saturates the subcutaneous fat beneath the patch. After 12–16 h, steady-state plasma fentanyl concentrations are reached, which are maintained for about 72 h. Fentanyl patches are currently available in 25, 50, 75, and 100 µg/h dosages. The bioavailability of transdermal fentanyl is very high, approximately 90%.

Advantages include:

+ it offers a non-invasive way of administering fentanyl to patients with stable pain in whom the 24-h opioid requirement has already been determined;
+ fentanyl is less constipating than morphine and this may offer a significant advantage to women with bowel dysfunction associated with abdomino-pelvic malignancy.

Disadvantages include:

+ Unsuitable for patients with uncontrolled pain.
+ Because of the slow depot formation and slow rise in plasma concentrations, this system is not suitable for patients with uncontrolled pain, as analgesia cannot be titrated rapidly.
+ Problems arise from conversion to fentanyl, as no clear protocols have been established. It has been suggested to use a conversion fentanyl-morphine ratio of 1:70–100. However, patients may still be under- or over-dosed and monitoring is essential until the correct dose has been established.

- Changes in rate of absorption with changes in body temperature—a fever-ish patient will absorb more fentanyl than one who is apyrexial because of vasodilatation in the skin.
- Slow offset of action once patch removed—fentanyl levels fall gradually once a patch is removed: this must be remembered if another drug is being started such as a subcutaneous opioid. It is important to give a reduced dose of the new drug for the first 12 h or so (with rescue medication available) and monitor the patient carefully.

The transmucosal/sublingual route

This is another route that may be useful in those patients unable to tolerate either oral drug therapy (e.g. nausea, vomiting, or dysphagia) or alternative parenteral routes such as lack of venous access.

Advantages include:

- sublingual venous drainage is systemic rather than portal and therefore hepatic first-pass elimination can be avoided;
- the transmucosal/sublingual route offers the potential for more rapid absorption and onset of action relative to the oral route.

Transmucosal route and breakthrough pain

This route (see above) is particularly useful for treating breakthrough pain, particularly when the pain is sudden in onset and short-lived, in which case an oral dose of opioid would take too long to have any beneficial effect.

Transmucosal fentanyl is the only medication that has been found to be a very useful tool in the management of breakthrough pain in cancer patients in different controlled studies—it also has a lower incidence of adverse effects than oral morphine. It is discussed in detail above in section on breakthrough pain.

Rectal route

This route may be a simple alternative when the oral route is not possible because of vomiting, obstruction, or altered consciousness.

Advantages include:

- independent of gastro-intestinal tract motility and rate of gastric emptying;
- simple;
- suitable for use at home by untrained carers or patients;
- staff do not need a high level of technical expertise to use it.

Disadvantages include:

- wide inter-individual variation in amount of drug drained from the rectum;
- absorption changed by surface area of rectum available for defecation;
- absorption disrupted by defecation or constipation;
- uncomfortable for prolonged use;
- cannot be used if patient has painful anal conditions such as fissures or inflamed haemorrhoids;
- does not bypass first-pass metabolism.

Dose equivalence Opioids are usually given at the oral dose.

Adjuvants

An important approach to a patient with pain that is poorly responsive to opioids is the co-administration of a non-opioid analgesic. There are a very large number of options.

Anti-depressants

Anti-depressants may improve depression, enhance sleep, and decrease the perception of pain. However, the analgesic effect of tricyclics is not directly related to anti-depressant activity. Common side-effects of tricyclic compounds include anti-muscarinic effects, such as dry mouth, impaired visual accommodation, urinary retention, and constipation, antihistaminic effects (sedation), and anti-alpha-adrenergic effects (orthostatic hypotension). The analgesic response, unlike an anti-depressant effect, is usually observed within 5 days. Alternative drugs with a lower incidence of side-effects should be considered in patients sensitive to the sedative, anticholinergic or hypotensive effects of amitriptyline. Despite the frequent use of amitriptyline in neuropathic cancer pain, its effectiveness has not been demonstrated appropriately in this context although good data is available for diabetic neuropathy for example.

Membrane stabilizers for neuropathic pain

It has been suggested that an anomaly in ion channels may play a role in the molecular mechanism of neuropathic pain. Systemic local anesthetics (e.g. mexiletine), carbamazepine, phenytoin, and sodium channel blockers, have been reported to relieve neuropathic pain states. Although the exact mechanism of these drugs is not known, they all inhibit the sodium channels of hyperactive and depolarized nerves, while not interfering with normal sensory function.

Although cancer patients with neuropathic pain have been reported to benefit from lignocaine, controlled studies failed to demonstrate any significant benefit. Although sodium channel-blocking agents are useful for the management of chronic neuropathic pain, no conclusive clinical study has statistically verified these observations in cancer pain.

Anticonvulsant drugs

Anticonvulsants, such as carbamazepine, phenytoin, valproate, and clonazepam, have been reported to relieve pain in numerous peripheral and central neuropathic pain conditions, although contradictory results have been found. Gabapentin is a promising drug as adjuvant to opioid analgesia for neuropathic cancer pain, although its superiority over amitriptyline has to be demonstrated.

Steroids in neuropathic pain

A number of studies have documented the positive effects of corticosteroids on various cancer-related symptoms, including pain, appetite, energy level, food consumption, general well-being, depression. However, most of the evidence for analgesic effects is anecdotal.

Clinicians sometimes use it when a tumour is thought to be pressing on a nerve with the intention of reducing peritumoural oedema and thereby reducing pressure on the nerve and possibly pain.

Bisphosphonates

Bisphosphonates have been found to potentiate the effects of analgesics in metastatic bone pain. Pamidronate, a potent bisphosphate, significantly reduced morbidity caused by bone metastases, including a 30–50% reduction in pain, impending pathological fractures, and the need for radiotherapy. Best results are obtained with doses of 60 or 90 mg pamidronate. This treatment is generally well-tolerated. Most investigators, primarily because of gastro-intestinal adverse events and the urgency of the situation, have preferred intra-venous administration of bisphosphonates. Recently, zomepiramate (zoledronic acid), a stronger bisphosphonate, has been used.

Ketamine

Ketamine is a non-competitive NMDA receptor blocker that exerts its primary effect when the NMDA-receptor-controlled ion channel has been opened by a nociceptive barrage—it should only be initiated on the advice/under supervision of a specialist. A synergistic effect between ketamine and opioids has been observed in cancer pain patients who had lost an analgesic response to high doses of morphine. Ketamine should be given at an initial starting dose of 100–150 mg daily, while the dose of opioids should be reduced by 50%, with the dose being titrated against the effect. The occurrence of adverse effects (such as hallucinations) may limit its analgesic efficacy.

Interventional procedures

Spinal route

A small number of patients may still not obtain adequate analgesia despite large systemic opioid doses and the use of adjuvant drugs, or they may suffer from uncontrollable side-effects such as nausea, vomiting, or sedation.

The goal of spinal opioid therapy is to place a small dose of an opioid and/or local anaesthetic close to the spinal opioid receptors located in the dorsal horn of the spinal cord to enhance analgesia and reduce systemic side-effects by decreasing the total daily opioid dose. Intrathecal opioid doses are one hundredth of the oral.

Epidural or intrathecal placement?

Use of this route to deliver opioids requires placing a catheter into the epidural or intrathecal (subarachnoid) space and using an external or implantable infusion pump to deliver the medication. Deciding between epidural vs. intrathecal placement or external vs. implantable pumps to deliver the opioid is based on multiple factors, including duration of therapy, type and location of the pain, disease extent and central nervous system involvement, opioid requirement, and individual experience. The daily epidural opioid requirement is approximately ten times that of intrathecal administration. Intrathecal opioid administration has the advantage of allowing a higher concentration of drug to be localized at the receptor site while minimizing systemic absorption, thus possibly decreasing drug-related side-effects. These are specialist techniques.

Choice of drug

Morphine and local anaesthetic combinations

Morphine remains the drug of choice for the spinal route, because of its relatively low lipid solubility resulting in a slow onset of action, but a long duration of analgesia when given via intermittent bolus. The starting dose is quite difficult to calculate and should take into consideration the previous opioid dose, the woman's age, and the mechanism underlying the pain. Adding a local anaesthetic (bupivacaine or ropivacaine) to morphine via the spinal route has been successful in providing good analgesia in patients whose pain was resistant to epidural morphine alone, despite high doses e.g. patients with neuropathic pain.

Morphine and clonidine in combination

Clonidine, an alpha-adrenergic agonist that acts at the dorsal horn of the spinal cord to produce analgesia, has been used in cancer patients in combination with epidural (or intrathecal) morphine infusions. There is some evidence to suggest that neuropathic pain may be somewhat more responsive to the combination of clonidine/morphine than to morphine alone, although orthostatic hypotension is of concern. This technique is still being evaluated.

Disadvantages include:

♦ high level of specialist knowledge and experience is needed to know when these techniques are most appropriate and for placement of the delivery system;

♦ introduction of infection: local infection may only require removal of catheter or delivery system but meningitis, epidural abscess and other CNS infections have been reported;

♦ the delivery system may not function properly;

♦ adverse drug reactions such as pruritus (opioids) or orthostatic hypertension (clonidine) are possible.[11]

Indications in pelvic malignancy

Spinal therapy can provide regional blockade for pelvic pain (nociceptive or neuropathic), incident neuropathic pain, or bony pain from metastatic disease in the vertebral column, pelvis, and lower limbs. These are all potentially difficult pains to manage on oral pharmacological therapy alone.

Hypogastric plexus block

It has been claimed that a superior hypogastric plexus block can be a highly effective method of controlling pelvic pain syndromes. It may not be completely effective however as pelvic tumours have a tendency to infiltrate somatic structures as well as nerves.

Pelvic cancers are often associated with myofascial involvement that causes somatic pain; pressure on the sciatic nerve frequently causes severe neuropathic pain. Therefore, the clinical picture is often mixed.

In conclusion, patients must be carefully selected for interventions such as a hypogastric plexus block or a sympathetic block for visceral pelvic pain. Retroperitoneal invasion may result in a limited spread of neurolytic solution and this may be another reason for failure or only partial success of a nerve block.

Cordotomy

A percutaneous cordotomy is the interruption of the ascending spinothalamic tract, usually at the cervical level. A percutaneous cervical cordotomy by radiofrequency has been used in patients with unilateral bone pain below the C5 dermatome.

The procedure is associated with potentially serious complications including:

- mirror pain, where a similar pain redevelops, sometimes with increased severity within weeks to months or the procedure;
- general fatigue;
- hemiparesis;
- respiratory failure—the phrenic nerve has its origins variably in C 3, 4, 5.

All these can cause a significant deterioration in the patient's performance status and quality of life, and are potentially hazardous.[4]

Summary

Pelvic pain syndromes in advanced pelvic malignancy commonly have a mixed aetiology requiring more than opioid therapy alone. The WHO pain ladder should be followed first and the oral route of opioid delivery should be the first choice. If the oral route cannot be used because of gastro-intestinal obstruction and/or severe nausea/vomiting, alternatives should be used, including transdermal, intravenous, or subcutaneous ones. As well as establishing an analgesic regimen, which provides continuous pain relief, analgesia should be provided for breakthrough pain, which needs to work within an appropriate period. If a rapid onset is needed, the subcutaneous, sublingual, or transmucosal routes (fentanyl lozenges) should be considered.

The spinal route could be used if the oral and other parenteral routes remain unsuccessful, despite trials with different opioids and the use of adjuvant drugs. Spinal analgesia may be most effective when opioids and local anaesthetics and/or clonidine are used in combination. Whatever route is used, administration of opioids to manage cancer pain requires knowledge of each drug's potency relative to morphine and bioavailability of the route chosen. Patients should be closely followed and doses titrated to minimize side-effects, whenever the opioid, route or dose is changed. Interventional procedures, such as neurolytic blocks, are seldom necessary and are associated with several problems. Their role has not still substantiated in controlled studies.

References

1 Rigor, B. M. (2000). Pelvic cancer pain. *J Surg Oncol*, **75**, 280–300.

2 Mercadante, S. and Portenoy, R. K. (2001). Opioid poorly responsive cancer pain. Part 2. Basic mechanisms that could shift dose-response for analgesia. *J Pain Symptom Managet*, **21**, 255–264.

3 Mercadante, S. (1999). Treatment and outcome of cancer pain in advanced cancer patients followed at home. *Cancer*, **85**,1849–1858.

4 Mercadante, S. (1997). Malignant bone pain: pathophysiology and treatment. *Pain*, **69**, 1–18.

5 Cervero, F. and Laird, J. M. A. (1999). Visceral pain. *Lancet*, **353**, 2145–2148.

6 Besson, J. M. (1999). The neurobiology of pain. *Lancet*, **353**, 1610–1615.

7 Mercadante, S. Casuccio, A., Agnello, A., Pumo, S., Kargar, J., and Garofalo, S. (1997). The analgesic effects of non-steroidal anti-inflammatory drugs (NSAIDs) in cancer pain due to somatic or visceral mechanism. *J Pain Symptom Manage*, **17**, 351–356.

8 Hanks, G. W. and the Expert Working group of the Research Network of the European Association for palliative care (2001). Morphine and alternative opioids in cancer pain: the EAPC recommendations. *Br J Cancer*, **84**, 587–593.

9 Portenoy, R. K., Payne, R., Coluzzi, P. *et al.* (1999). Oral transmucosal fentanyl citrate (OTFC) for the treatment of breakthrough pain in cancer patients: a controlled dose titration study. *Pain*, **79**, 303–312.

10 Bruera, E., Pereira, J., Watanabe, M., Belzile, M., Kuehn, N., and Hanson, J. (1996). A retrospective comparison of dose ratios between methadone, hydromorphone and morphine. *Cancer*, **78**, 852–857.

11 Mercadante, S. (1999). Problems of long-term spinal opioid treatment in advanced cancer patients. *Pain*, **79**, 1–13.

Chapter 5

The management of odours and discharges in gynaecological cancer

Teresa Tate

Introduction

Society still imposes rigid rules on some areas of an individual's behaviour, particularly in aspects of personal hygiene. Among these are the expectations that people will not smell unpleasantly and that discharges of any sort from the body will not be offensive and will be concealed. Any person who develops a problem of odour or discharge becomes stigmatized by a sense of general disgust, which may be barely concealed even by close family members. The onset of these symptoms in the context of a diagnosis of cancer carries a complex significance for the patient, impacting on her sense of worth and self as a social being and on her own body image, as well as very specifically re-inforcing the fact of ill-health.

Discharges in the setting of a patient with gynaecological cancer are usually due to the breakdown of tissue resulting in loss of fluid either from a necrotic mass of cells or from erosion into a hollow viscus, particularly the bowel or the urinary tract. Odour from these ulcerated areas is caused by the fluid itself or by added infection.

In simple terms, management is aimed at treating infection, and reducing and confining fluid loss. Traditionally these problems have been the concern of nurses, and the nursing literature contains a number of articles describing individual interventions, but there is very little formal trial evidence to guide clinical decision-making. This chapter will address the management of odours and discharges directly related to cancer or the treatment of cancer, but many of the principles discussed may be applied to the management of benign lesions, such as pressure-area breakdown, which are also common in women with advanced gynaecological cancer.

Evidence

Much of the literature concerns the management of cutaneous lesions, particularly in breast cancer, and little is written about other tumours. It is not always possible to extrapolate management advice to internal ulcerating areas. The advice in this chapter has drawn on clinical experience and the few comparative trials available. These difficult problems are unique to each patient, in both the physical and psychosocial sense,[1] and individualized treatment plans must be developed from the broad guidance suggested here.

Patients at risk

Odours and discharges develop in women with gynaecological cancer in circumstances that result in a tumour mass eroding through the epithelium to the surface or through its mucosal surrounding into another organ or body cavity. This may occur:

- following surgical resection when the excision margins are close or microscopic tumour has been cut through;

- following radiation or chemotherapy when tumour persists or recurs;

- with superficial nodal disease in the groin, which is at particular risk of eroding the skin. These examples of tumour directly eroding outside the body will result in discharge and odour, as these lesions very easily become infected often with anaerobes such as bacteroides.

Discharges can also occur when enterocutaneous fistulae develop from benign or malignant causes (see Chapter 6).

- In advanced ovarian cancer, fistulae from the small or large bowel may follow the initial debulking surgical procedure, especially if bowel resection has been necessary.

- Local pelvic recurrences, particularly of carcinoma of the cervix, can result in erosion of the urethra, bladder or lower portion of the ureters.

The discharged material will be faecal fluid or urine, rather than identifiable necrotic tumour, but may still be very offensive and difficult to manage.

Discharges containing or composed of blood may not be significantly offensive, but are particularly frightening for the patient and concerning for the clinician.

Assessment

The approach taken to the patient complaining of an odour or discharge should be no different to any other assessment in medical practice and is based on fundamental principles. Making the best possible diagnosis of the cause of the problem, and the best possible assessment of the effect of the symptom on the patient, should result in the best possible treatment plan being developed.

History

A careful history should be taken with a particular emphasis on any observations the patient may have made of events or activities that exacerbate or relieve the problem. Review of any operation notes or radiation treatment records, combined with the patient's story, may be sufficient to make a pathological diagnosis in many cases. Ask about:

- rate of change of size of the lesion;
- volume and nature of discharge, especially to differentiate urine or faeces;
- whether there is bleeding;
- pain and response to analgesics (see Chapter 4).

Physical examination

This is an essential part of the diagnostic process, but may be difficult for both patient and clinician when the lesion is particularly offensive. It is usually helpful to the patient to acknowledge the unpleasant odour, rather than to pretend not to have noticed it. This will be an opportunity to reassure the patient that you will be able to suggest strategies for improving the smell. Look for:

- size of the lesion and relationship to other structures;
- volume and nature of discharge, is a fistula present?;
- potential for treatment, e.g. ease of resectability;
- ease of containment.

Imaging

This may be required if the full extent of the lesion is not understood at the end of the history taking and examination. As in all situations when the intention of treatment is palliation of a symptom, sophisticated investigations should not be withheld, provided the patient is fit enough, if it is believed that that investigation will assist in making the diagnosis.

Review previous imaging:

- cross-sectional images will define tumour masses and spatial relationships;
- consider a fistulogram to define extent of internal track.

Other investigations:

- microbiological screen;
- methylene blue dye test, if a vesicovaginal fistula is suspected;
- biopsy to distinguish between tumour and radiation necrosis.

Psychological assessment

This is an important part of the initial evaluation, as the symptoms may be causing the patient significant distress. Many women go to extraordinary lengths to conceal such problems as far as possible and to invent methods of covering, which may take hours of their time each day. They may admit to having completely altered their lifestyle, to being unable to leave the house or to engage in any form of social activity, or any family intimacy such as cuddling their grandchildren. These forced changes in behaviour often compound an already existing belief that their role as a feminine and sexual being has been taken away by the diagnosis and treatment of a gynaecological cancer (see Chapter 8)

> It is not necessary for any clinician to have formal counselling skill training to begin to acknowledge and explore the woman's feelings in relation to these problems. It may be helpful to involve a specialist nurse at this stage, if the patient does not already have access to such a service.

Management

Symptoms such as odour or discharge should not be dismissed as unimportant, but must be managed as part of an integrated plan for the palliative care for the patient, since they most frequently reflect advancing cancer.[2, 3] It is, however, important to establish, with as much certainty as possible, if there is a benign cause for the symptom. This is clearly important for the patient and the clinician in understanding the prognosis, and also for determining the management plan. The treatment plan required to manage pelvic radiation necrosis is as complex as that which will be required for recurrent tumour, but clearly has an entirely different emphasis.

The focus should be on improving the patient's quality of life. A multi-professional assessment is valuable, especially since, in the absence of a large evidence base, the skills and experience of individual clinicians can contribute enormously to an appropriate plan.

> It can be helpful to use the patient's estimated prognosis as a guide. Initially consider the most radical or aggressive approaches and then, as these are judged inappropriate, move to increasingly palliative treatments.

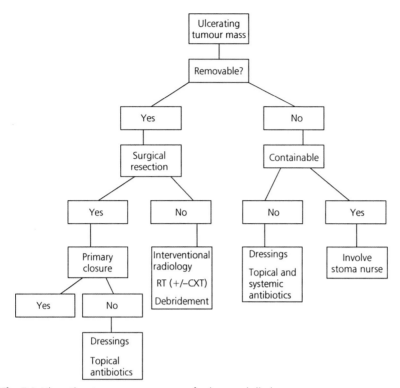

Fig. 5.1 Ulcerating tumours as a cause of odour and discharge.

Figure 5.1 suggests an approach to the management of an ulcerating cuta-neous or mucosal tumour mass. General medical and nursing measures for the care of the woman are of course essential. These include improvement in nutrition, attention to bowel and bladder function, and importantly, optimal pain management.

Removable tumour mass

In situations when the overall tumour burden is low and the woman's prognosis is judged to be months or more, it is appropriate to consider treatments that can ablate the tumour:

- if the mass cannot be surgically removed, it may be possible to achieve control using radiation or chemotherapy;
- selective interventional radiology techniques that occlude the tumour cir-culation may be useful, particularly if the lesion is bleeding (see below);

- debridement of the mass by various techniques, e.g. laser, cryosurgery, can significantly improve odour and discharge.

Cutaneous ulceration

The intended management plan must be as compatible as possible with the woman's intended level of activity and her normal style of clothing. Nursing access to some lesions, for example in the crease of the groin, may be difficult in frail and elderly patients with osteoarthritis of the hips. Holding dressings in place if the patient is mobile may also present difficulties.

- keep the affected area as cool as possible (NB nursing ill patients on temperature maintained specialist beds may result in an increase in odour);
- regular (3–4 times daily) irrigation with normal saline and dressing changes;
- odour and discharge can be reduced by topical de-sloughing agents;
- exudate can be reduced by high absorbency dressings and foams;
- stoma bags can be individually tailored to cover the area;
- topical metronidazole gel 0.8% will reduce anaerobic infection and odour;[4]
- charcoal-impregnated coverings will contain odour;
- combination dressings are available that have de-sloughing and absorbent properties and also contain charcoal.

Mucosal and internal ulceration

It will not be possible to apply dressings directly to some lesions, e.g. in the vagina. The aims of treatment are the same, but must be achieved more indirectly:

- regular douching with normal saline;
- tampons will absorb discharge;
- treat infections, e.g. candida, with optimal dose local and/or oral therapy;
- oral metronidazole 400 mg three times daily for 7 days to reduce odour;
- charcoal-impregnated dressings worn inside loose fitting cotton underpants will contain odour.

Bleeding from an ulcerated tumour

Sero-sanginous fluid is commonly lost from tumour ulcers and has no sinister significance. However, frank bleeding may occur from a mass that may be in close proximity to a blood vessel, or may itself be very vascular.

- Small volume oozing can be controlled by pressure and haemostatic dressings.
- Infection precipitating bleeding should be treated.
- Radiotherapy will reduce tumour-related bleeding.
- Clotting abnormalities may be corrected.
- Oral tranexamic acid 1000–1500 mg two to three times daily. (15–25 mg/kg body wt three times daily).
- If there is a risk of a significant bleed from the tumour, it is essential that a management plan is discussed, agreed, and recorded. A decision about whether the patient is involved in a detailed discussion of the possibility of a fatal bleed, should be made on an individual basis. The principles of the woman's right to information and to make choices about her treatment should be remembered.
- Decisions should be made about transfusion if bleeding persists and about the extent of resuscitation to be undertaken if an acute large haemorrhage occurs. These are complex decisions that should be made on an individual basis and should involve input from all members of the multidisciplinary team.

Enterovaginal or vesicovaginal fistulae as a cause of odour and discharge

The loss of continence caused by fistulae into the vagina is a most distressing and undignified symptom for a woman to suffer. It is essential that, in every case, consideration is given to restoring control if possible.

- The most radical management approach, suitable only for a small minority of carefully assessed patients, is a palliative pelvic exenteration, which can result in a substantial improvement in quality of life and will also resect all microscopically demonstrated tumour.
- For most relatively fit patients able to tolerate a general anaesthetic, diverting surgery is the most effective way to contain the fluid loss. Although loop colostomies may be performed more quickly, there is a higher risk of stomal recurrence. There is little difference in early morbidity or survival between end or loop colostomies.
- Urinary diversion may be achieved by the formation of a continent conduit or by the insertion of bilateral nephrostomy tubes.
- Diversion will be necessary to allow a benign fistula to heal.

The choice of surgical procedure will be guided by the surgeon's assessment of technical feasibility and the fitness of the patient, but most importantly by the patient's own assessment of the value and acceptability of the predicted outcome of the intervention.

For those patients who are too unfit, or who decide against a surgical procedure, meticulous assistance with skin care and local hygiene is required.

- depending on the site of the fistula, a urethral or supra pubic catheter will contain the urine;
- barrier cream will protect the skin;
- laxatives containing danthron should be stopped as this damages the skin;
- women have different preferences about wearing pads—various sizes should be available.

Enterocutaneous fisulae as a cause of odour and discharge

These fistulae most commonly develop between the small bowel and a surgical incision line. The volume of faecal fluid output may be 2–3 l/day and the patient may become dehydrated quickly.

- Management is aimed at containing the fluid. The advice of an experienced stoma nurse is vital as these wounds may extend and enlarge irregularly. They are often sited over an uneven area of skin, which causes difficulties with adhesion and in achieving a water tight base for a stoma bag.
- The surrounding skin needs protection from the corrosive ileal fluid with a barrier cream.
- The output of fluid from the fistula can be reduced in volume using somatostatin analogues, e.g. octreotide 100 μg three times daily by subcutaneous injection, which can be increased every 48 h if there is no obvious response. Current evidence suggests that no further response will be achieved by increasing the daily total dose above 1200 μg. There are long-acting preparations that are suitable in a stable, chronic situation (see Chapter 7).
- Reducing the flow through a fistulous track will encourage healing if the cause is benign.

General measures

The odour of a necrotic, infected tumour mass is characteristic, cloying, pervasive, and often very over-powering. In addition to the social and psychological effects already mentioned, the smell may have more direct effects. Many women complain of anorexia and alteration of the sensation of taste or persistent nausea. These symptoms are also sometimes suffered by other members of the household and those professional carers who attend the patient. Healthcare workers often complain that they take the smell away with them when they leave the patient.

In addition to all the specific treatments suggested above, there are some useful measures which can improve the local environment:

◆ frequent changes of clothing and bed linen;

◆ circulation of air if the space is confined;

◆ aroma therapy burners or atomisers, using citrus oils, particularly grapefruit;

◆ commercially available domestic air-freshening aerosols may be used, but often work by providing another scent, which can be as unacceptable to the patient and her carers;

◆ small portable air filters can be helpful, but are frequently noisy, and effective only in small spaces.

Our sense and appreciation of smell is known to influence many aspects of our lives; affecting our mood, how hard we concentrate, and even spend money. It is clear that a persisting unpleasant odour can have a profound effect on any woman who develops a fungating tumour. It is incumbent on all clinicians to make every possible effort to reduce the impact of the problem for the patient and her family.

References

1   Anonymous (2000). Fungating wounds. In *The Royal Marsden Hospital Manual of Clinical Nursing Procedures*, 5th edn (Mallett, J. and Dougherty, L. eds), pp. 693–697. Blackwell, Oxford.

2   Ivetic, O. and Lyne, P. A. (1990). Fungating and ulcerating malignant lesions: a review of the literature. *J Adv Nurs*, 15(1), 83–88.

3   Haisfield-Wolfe, M. E. and Rund, C. (1997). Malignant cutaneous wounds: a management protocol. *Ostomy Wound Manage*, 43(1), 56–60.

4   Finlay, I. G., Bowszyc, J., Ramlau, C., and Gwiezdzinski, Z. (1996). The effect of topical 0.75% metronidazole gel on malodorous cutaneous ulcers. *J Pain Symptom Manage*, 11(3), 158–162.

Chapter 6

The management of fistulae

Robin Crawford

Introduction

Fistulae can be a significant problem for the patient dying from gynaecological cancer. A fistula developing as a complication of treatment (surgical or radiotherapeutic) in a patient undergoing curative therapy can usually be tackled aggressively with the aim of restoring function and this is usually successful. The palliative care patient with advanced disease is doubly disadvantaged as the fistula will remind her of the incurable nature of her condition and, in addition, such patients are often not fit to undergo significant surgical intervention to attempt repair. The symptoms caused by a fistula can be managed in several ways in order to improve the quality of life for the patient for the remainder of her days. The methods chosen to do this usually depend on the experience of the local clinical team as there is very little evidence available on how to control the symptoms resulting from this problem.

Summary of evidence available

Most of the information relating to the management of palliative care patients with fistulae is anecdotal or discussed in a very general manner in textbooks. This is because each patient with advanced disease has an individual set of circumstances and goals, which makes a uniform management plan difficult. In a cancer centre, there may only be a handful of patients a year requiring specialized input for this condition and, therefore, experience is gained only over a long period of time. During this period, data collection may be sparse, treatments (both medical and surgical) and the attitudes to intervention may change because the evidence-base increases and because over that time some 'fashionable' treatments prove to have little value.

This chapter is not referenced but it is drawn from experience working in several cancer centres.

Background

A fistula is a track linking two epithelial surfaces. Fistulae occur in women with malignant disease for a variety of reasons and can be classified by cause, the volume and the sort of output from them, the size of the defect, and anatomical site. Fistulae can be the result of treatment or due to disease progression.

The common types of fistulae involve the vagina. Other fistulae track from the gastro-intestinal tract to the skin, often discharging through a wound or a drain site. On occasions, fistulae can develop between organs within the abdominal cavity, e.g. an entero-vesical fistula. This type of fistula will lead to pneumaturia, passage of faeculant urine, and infection. It is possible for a patient to have multiple fistulae such as a combined entero-colo-vaginal fistula or a urethral-vesico-vaginal fistula. Combined urinary fistulae are present in 20% of cases.

The most common causes of fistulae are surgery or radiotherapy given as primary treatment.

Fistulae following surgery

These will be dealt with as a post-operative complication. Direct surgical injury from an inappropriately placed suture or a diathermy burn causing a hole or necrosis is seen typically following the primary surgery and develops in the first 5–7 days post-operatively. Fistulae resulting from ischaemic damage are usually apparent in the 6 weeks following surgery. The risk of developing a fistula is between 0.5% and 6% depending on the group of patients reported. Usually a fistula rate of <1% would be considered acceptable for primary treatment at a good centre. The prognosis for an uncomplicated post-surgical fistula is good.

Fistulae relating to radiotherapy

These develop at different rates: those affecting the bowel occur between 6 and 18 months after the end of treatment, and those affecting the bladder between 18 and 48 months after treatment. The majority of serious radiotherapy complications have occurred within 5 years of the end of treatment but there is a small but continuous risk of complications occurring as long as 20 years afterwards. Due to the nature of radiotherapy change, stricture formation and later fistula formation can occur. This is due to radiotherapy damage to the small vessels leading to endarteritis obliterans.

Fistulae in patients receiving palliative care

Patients within the sphere of palliative care may have fistulae resulting from recurrent disease, infection, or tissue necrosis. Fistulae can develop when the natural flow of the secretions or fluids within a viscus is blocked. Bowel obstruction may resolve by the development of a fistula, which allows drainage of the blocked contents.

The size of defect can be large or small. The larger fistulae can be complex with involvement of rectum, bladder, urethra, and small bowel with the vagina (also known as a cloaca) or a large area of skin with multiple fistula tracts through a wound. These large defects are more difficult to manage than the single small fistula, which is managed in a similar way to a standard stoma. Fistulae that follow radiation therapy are often complex, involving discharge of urine, faeces, and even tissue from necrotic tumour.

Fistuale in patients with advanced ovarian cancer

A fistula would be a very unusual primary presentation of ovarian cancer but a fistula may develop through the abdominal or vaginal incisions following primary surgery. The likelihood of a fistula is increased if there is a significant amount of bowel surgery. The role of aggressive debulking in the primary surgical procedure has not been clearly defined and even when the surgery involving bowel resection and anastomosis is performed to the highest standard, there is still a risk of anastomotic leak which can lead to fistula formation.

History

The typical history of a vaginal fistula is of a persistent continuous discharge, which is either watery (vesico- or uretero-vaginal fistula) or faeculant (recto- or entero-vaginal fistula). The onset of incontinence of urine of the sort where the woman is wet all the time is very suggestive of vesico-vaginal fistula. Pneumaturia or passing flatus when micturating is the classic sign of a colo-vesical fistula. A brown vaginal discharge may consist of blood, tumour, or faecal material. Some women give a clear history of increasing abdominal pain and feeling unwell, which is then associated with the sudden passage of stool or flatus per vaginum, followed by a general improvement and then a new symptom of passing altered, increased, and foul vaginal discharge. This suggests an obstruction or collection that has settled by fistulation. The type of material draining from the fistula can help determine its site. A low-volume smelly discharge is more likely to be colonic in origin (e.g. colo-cutaneous or colo-vaginal). A high-volume non-smelly but corrosive type of effluent is more typical of a small bowel fistula (e.g. ileo-cutaneous)—these tend to have higher volumes of discharge.

Examination

Examination may reveal recurrent tumour. The presence of a defect (the fistula) on vaginal examination is sometimes detectable. The defect on the abdominal wall is usually clear with an entero-cutaneous fistula. Sometimes these may present as an abscess or subcutaneous mass with fluctuant contents; suspicion of an underlying fistula should always be raised in this circumstance. Microbiological culture of the discharge/pus may reveal gut organisms suggestive of a connection with the GI tract.

Possible investigations

Historically, the investigation of fistulae into the vagina included examination under anaesthesia with swabs in the vagina and coloured fluid instilled into the bladder or rectum.

Nowadays, the value of good radiological support cannot be overemphasized. Liaison with the radiologist will help determine the site of the fistula. The radiologist requires information on the clinical stage of the disease, clinical suspicion about the origin of the fistula, previous surgery (what has been removed and what is still present), and other therapy for the disease such as radiotherapy. MRI can be very useful in determining the origin and the extent of the fistula in the pelvis, as it can show the abnormal fluid-filled track. Other imaging of the abdomen may be appropriate, especially if surgical correction is required. This is to ensure that there is no distal obstruction to the fistula or multiple fistulae, which are present in 20% of cases.

Endoscopic examination, including cystoscopy or rigid/flexible sigmoidoscopy, can be helpful in assessing the bladder, rectum, and sigmoid colon. It is important to detect the presence of recurrent tumour. An examination under anaesthetic allows appreciation of the extent of the fistula without discomfort for the patient and biopsies can be taken to exclude recurrent disease. Caution should be exercised when taking biopsies in an irradiated field, as this can lead to wounds that do not, or which are slow to, heal.

Haematological and biochemical assessment is often helpful to assess the patient's general well-being, including detecting anaemia and/or renal impairment.

Assessment

The decision on whether to operate on a patient with advancing disease and a fistula is not an easy one. A simple colostomy may not be possible because of disease affecting the rest of the bowel (especially in ovarian cancer) and the presence of a complex fistula involving different levels of the GI tract. The formation of the stoma can precipitate disease fungating onto the abdominal wall.

Who can help?

A multidisciplinary approach is required for the management of fistulae in women with advanced malignancy.

Detection of the fistula is central to psychological as well as physical treatment, as the symptoms may be considered bizarre and are frightening as well as stigmatizing. The smell of faecal or urinary incontinence, or the discomfort caused by tissue damage resulting from an ileal fistula, are distressing. The initial approach should be an attempt to alleviate the symptoms and to assess the significance of the fistula for the woman in relation to her overall well-being. Radiological investigation (see below) is then required both to delineate the fistula accurately and to determine whether there is tumour recurrence present. The management of the fistula does depend on the remaining life-expectancy. A surgical approach with formation of stomas may be appropriate in a patient with a reasonable life-expectancy but may be wholly inappropriate for a woman with only weeks to live. Discussion between the woman, her carers, and the physicians will need to be frank and two-way, so that the final decision made about surgical treatment or other care is as good as possible.

Psychological support for these women is important. Not only is the fistula a constant reminder of the recurrent disease but the uncontrolled loss of bodily fluids, often associated with a foul smell, is degrading. Positive action to alleviate symptoms, as well as an explanation of the causes and the significance of the fistula, are helpful for the patient and her carers. (See Chapter 5.)

Management

Physical methods

The symptoms from a vaginal fistula may be helped by a tampon giving temporary relief, which allows the woman to mobilize and socialize for short time-periods. A urethral catheter may help in reducing the loss by keeping the bladder empty and thereby improving quality of life, ease of nursing, and give some freedom from the wetness and smell of the urinary loss. Occasionally, occluding the vagina with a large Foley catheter (20 French guage with a large balloon) can also give temporary relief from fluid loss from the vagina. It works by forming a seal lower in the vagina whilst the drainage channel allows for the removal of the urine or diarrhoea. A leg bag connected to the catheter can conceal the collecting device under clothing.

Other devices for occluding the vagina have been described and their availability depends on local resources. Modified menstrual collecting devices, methyl methacrylate, and alginate-shaped vaginal moulds have been reported in the literature to tamponade the vagina and allow controlled drainage of the effluent.

Ureteric and colonic stents

In the presence of a ureteric fistula, stent insertion may may provide a conduit allowing flow along the natural pathway into the bladder and so provide symptom relief.

Endoscopic stenting of the colon has been reported with variable results in the palliation of bowel obstruction and, although not reported in the literature, it may in theory be useful in the management of a fistula as well.

Other measures

Barrier creams can be useful to protect the skin from the effect of the fistula output. The use of a stoma appliance may allow collection of the effluent in a clean, efficient manner. Advice from the specialist stoma nurse can usually result in an effective seal around a cutaneous fistula. Low-pressure drainage, with an occlusive dressing covering the defect, may allow clean nursing and avoid the problems of odour. Suction drainage of a fistula will maintain its integrity and inhibit any spontaneous closure.

Drug therapy

With a low recto-vaginal fistula, the output can be managed in a similar way to a stoma. The use of codeine phosphate or other antimotility agents, such as loperamide, may promote a more solid stool consistency enabling it to be removed more easily. Alternatively, a bulking agent such as ispaghula may be helpful in reducing the loss from the defect, so that the woman may then be able to function without any loss for several hours. Enteric fistulae may be difficult to manage because of their high output. Octreotide and/or hyoscine butylbromide may be needed to reduce the flow of secretions from such fistulae.

The standard management of a small bowel fistula includes parenteral nutrition reducing the bowel activity, but the decision to do this must be made carefully. There are occasions when parenteral nutrition is started and it then becomes obvious that there is no rapid resolution to the clinical problem. The withdrawal of the parenteral nutrition then becomes tantamount to withdrawing active intervention and can be fraught for patient, carers, and the medical staff. Hence there is a reticence to use parenteral nutrition without a clearly defined time parameter for observing an objective response, e.g. a 2-week attempt to see whether the fistula closes spontaneously.

Surgical approaches

Whilst a surgical approach will almost always correct the uncontrolled loss of faeces or urine with a stoma or diversion, not all patients will opt for this, nor will all patients be fit enough for this intervention.

Fistulae following surgery for primary treatment of the tumour

Most of these patients are in a good nutritional state and their tissues have not been irradiated. Vesico- or uretero-vaginal fistulae are the most common, and they can be treated by prolonged bladder drainage or ureteral stenting. This will usually allow healing to take place without recourse to further surgery but occasionally, surgical repair is required. It is important to leave at least eight weeks between the initial causative operation and the operative repair to allow infection, oedema, and inflammation to settle. In the UK, the vesico-vaginal fistula is usually repaired transabdominally by urologists, as the overall number of fistulae seen is low. There are some proponents of a vaginal approach for low fistulae but this is seldom appropriate when the aetiology is malignant. The most important factor governing the success of the procedure is that the clinician has experience of this type of surgery, whether using a vaginal or an abdominal approach. Interposition of vascularized tissue is helpful to separate the suture lines of the repair and allows better healing. The omentum is usually used for the transabdominal approach and the Martius graft from the labial fat pad for the transvaginal repair. The results of repair are usually excellent in this group of patients.

Good surgical technique, antibiotic prophylaxis and careful patient selection can reduce the likelihood of fistula formation. Increasingly, gynaecological oncology surgeons are operating in a non-irradiated field, in patients with early disease and a good nutritional and performance status, and perhaps performing less radical surgery. For example, in patients with cervical cancer most centres in the UK are operating on patients with smaller cancers using a less extensive type 2 Routledge radical hysterectomy procedure, which in turn leads to a smaller risk of fistula formation.

Fistulae in patients with advanced disease

These are commonly rectal and enteric fistulae, which are more problematic. A small rectal fistula may be managed by using an agent to bulk the patient's stool, which may lead to a minimal amount of soiling, which is often acceptable to the patient. Definitive management requires diversion of the faecal stream with a stoma, then repair of the fistula at a later date. In the palliative setting it is important to consider a holistic approach rather than just focus on the defect, as the patient may only have time or be fit enough for the first stage of the procedure (diversion). A delayed repair is important as it allows the inflammation and infection to settle, as well enabling the woman to return home after an unexpected prolonged initial hospital stay. The covering stoma is then closed some months after the repair has been performed and has been shown to be intact using radiological investigations.

Operating in a patient who has been irradiated can lead to a ten-fold increase in fistulae. However, surgery following radiotherapy treatment is relatively rare—an example would be exenteration for a central pelvic recurrence of cervical cancer after primary therapy. Although in some series the 5-year survival after surgery is as high as 50%, there is also a high rate of fistula formation (10–20%). As discussed in a previous section, prolonged drainage of the fistula (which has to be accompanied by the use of parenteral nutrition for the patient) can allow healing to occur in a number of cases without recourse to further surgery. Where more surgery is required, it is often associated with horrendous complications. It is therefore vital that the patient and her carers should share making the decision, as often there are no really acceptable solutions.

Recto-vaginal fistula

These can be repaired surgically. If the patient is reasonably fit, a defunctioning colostomy (either an end colostomy or a loop colostomy) can be performed easily. An end colostomy is easier to manage when the application of the stoma device is considered. A colostomy gives good control of the fistula by diverting the faecal flow, allowing resolution of symptoms (uncontrolled loss, soiling, and odour). However, the patient will have to undergo a surgical procedure under general anaesthetic. The additional problems for the dying patient are that they will have a new stoma that will new require care and support. Although care for the stoma may be straightforward, in a dying patient, it may represent further loss of her independence because she will need help to manage the stoma initially. The stoma will also be a visible reminder of her impending death.

Entero-vaginal fistula

Options for an entero-vaginal fistula repair include excision of the fistulated section, internal bypass (entero-colic bypass), or ileostomy. Before embarking on a surgical solution, it is important to delineate where the fistula is within the small bowel. It is unusual in the palliative setting to resect and re-anastomose the fistulated segment, as the operative procedure is more prolonged and the disease in such patients is frequently widespread. Occasionally, a bypass of the fistula segment can be performed, which is of course the better outcome as it avoids a stoma. It is important to know that the colon is not obstructed before the ileo-colic bypass is performed. Unfortunately, with advanced disease, it is unusual to have only one area of disease allowing an internal bypass. Entero-vaginal fistulae can also be managed by ileostomy, however, these fistule often have a high output and can leave the patient quite dehydrated. The management of a high-output stoma requires good nursing and continuing support to ensure there is no leakage from the bag.

Urinary fistulae

Urinary fistulae can be corrected by an ileal conduit. However, this may be difficult if there has been extensive radiation and recurrent disease. The use of nephrostomy is not recommended as the drainage does not remove all the fluid and is temporary. A ureteral fistula may close or be significantly reduced by the insertion of a stent. This may be done transvesically or via a nephrostomy. Closure of a ureteric fistula may require a cross-over to the other ureter or the use of a piece of ileum to bridge the damaged portion, often connecting this straight into the bladder. A vesico-vaginal fistula may be corrected by an ileal conduit. It needs to be remembered that all these procedures are major operations for a woman in the palliative stages of her disease and, if the patient has a conduit, she will then also have to manage the stoma bag. On the other hand, the formation of an ileal conduit may be the safest surgical treatment, especially with extensive pelvic radiotherapy.

A rarely used alternative management is to use the rectum as a reservoir for the urine. By closing the vagina distal to the fistula (colpocleisis) and creating an artificial connection to the rectum from the vagina (rectal fenestration), the fistula is diverted into the continent rectum. This relies on the presence of a functioning anal sphincter, which can be tested by instilling 500–1000 ml of warm saline into the rectum and checking that the woman is continent. If she can hold the test volume, then it may be appropriate to use the rectum as a reservoir for her urine. The advantage for this procedure is that it may be performed vaginally resulting in a smaller operation with a quicker recovery time and no stoma.

Malignant fluid collections

The management of discharging infected cysts or malignant fluid collections, such as a lymphocysts, can be difficult. These are not strictly fistulae but they are approached in a similar fashion to cutaneous fistulae, with the aim of resolving the symptoms at the same time as finding out whether definitive management of the underlying problem is possible.

Conclusion

The presence of gynaecological fistulae in palliative care is rare. Management is aimed at providing the woman with relief from the uncontrolled loss of malodourous or corrosive fluids, and it is essential that sustaining and improving quality of life are the central aims of any treatment the patient needs to understand and choose from the treatment options available in consultation with her surgeon and other medical advisors.

Chapter 7

The management of bowel obstruction in advanced gynaecological malignancy

Doreen Oneschuk

Incidence and general features

Malignant bowel obstruction (MBO) is a common complication in patients with ovarian cancer, colorectal cancer, and other malignancies involving the pelvis. Some 25–42% of patients with advanced ovarian carcinoma develop obstruction, but it rarely occurs with endometrial cancer and MBO in patients with cervical cancer is usually caused by post-irradiation fibrosis.

Pathological mechanisms involved in the development of malignant bowel obstruction include:

1. A mechanical obstruction from an extrinsic occlusion of the bowel lumen.
2. An intraluminal occlusion of the lumen.
3. A luminal obstruction resulting from tumour growth from within the bowel wall.
4. An adynamic ileus or other intestinal motility disorder. A motility disorder is a functional obstruction, i.e. there is no occlusion of the bowel lumen. Motility disorders cannot be distinguished from luminal obstruction by their clinical features alone.[1–6]

It is important to remember that in ovarian cancer, occlusion and motility disorders often co-exist and obstruction may occur at many sites. Malignant bowel obstruction is often multi-factorial in advanced disease—functional obstruction is common in ovarian cancer because tumour often infiltrates the bowel wall or mesentery affecting the nerve supply and muscle function.

Bowel obstruction can also result from non-malignant causes—these include:

- adhesions;
- post-irradiation bowel damage;
- inflammatory bowel disease;
- hernias.

Bowel obstruction may be:

- intermittent or permanent;
- at single or multiple sites.

Even apparently 'complete' bowel obstruction can resolve spontaneously and the clinical course is unpredictable.

Editor's note: This clinical unpredictability and the multiple etiologies of bowel obstruction in advanced cancer makes the terms 'acute', 'subacute', 'incomplete', and 'partial' obstruction very inexact and many authorities think it would be better not to qualify the term 'obstruction'. The description of bowel obstruction as acute/subacute or partial or complete is very common but when using these descriptions the clinician needs to remember that they are not predicative of clinical course, nor are they associated with a particular aetiology.

The small bowel is more commonly affected than the large bowel, but both may be simultaneously involved, especially in ovarian cancer. About 60% of cases of obstruction occur in the small bowel and are secondary to extrinsic compression. Most patients with intestinal obstruction and ovarian cancer will live less than one year, the majority dying within 6 months of presenting with this complication.[1, 5]

Sources of evidence

Most of the evidence about bowel obstruction is derived from retrospective or pilot studies. The methodology in many of the studies is of poor quality—statistical analysis and outcome measures (e.g. quality of life and symptom control) are often lacking.

Pathophysiology

The pathophysiology of malignant bowel obstruction can be considered as a pernicious cycle of abdominal distention leading to intestinal fluid secretion and increased peristalsis. Malignant bowel obstruction begins with a simple blockage and intestinal distention. As luminal contents accumulate, intestinal fluid secretion is stimulated, further distending the bowel wall and obstructing

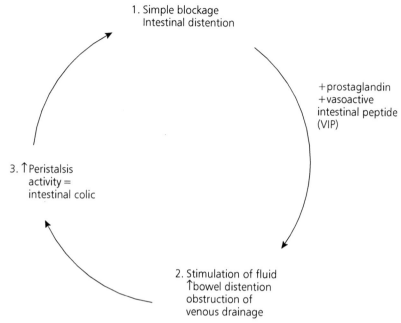

Fig. 7.1 Cycle of distension–intestinal secretion–peristalsis.

venous drainage in the affected segment of bowel. Simultaneously, intermittent peristaltic activity occurs in an attempt to surmount the obstruction. Prostaglandin and vasoactive intestinal peptide (VIP) secretion further enhance intestinal fluid secretion.[3, 4]

Assessment and Clinical Features

Key points in the history

Assess the presence, quality and intensity of the following symptoms:

- abdominal pain—may be diffuse, dull and achy; and constant;
- abdominal pain—cramping, colicky and intermittent.

Both sorts of abdominal pain can occur in the same episode of obstruction.

- nausea;
- emesis—nausea and vomiting must be separately assessed.
- the passage of flatus;
- stool—both diarrhoea and constipation are possible in bowel obstruction;
- loss of appetite;
- the presence of borborygmi.

A numerical analogue scale (i.e. score of 1–10) is a useful way of assessing the intensity of symptoms and when consistently recorded allows continuity of care when medical and nursing staff change shifts.

Abdominal pain

Continuous abdominal pain is the most common symptom and is caused by intra-abdominal tumor. Intermittent colic may occur when superimposed intestinal segmental activity occurs in attempts to surmount the obstacle in the bowel. The colicky pain of large bowel obstruction tends to be deeper and occurs at longer intervals. The constant pain of a pelvic tumour in large bowel obstruction can be very severe.

Vomiting

This develops early (and is copious) in gastric, duodenal, and small bowel obstruction: it tends to occur later in the course of large bowel obstruction when facealent vomiting may occur. Facealent vomiting also occurs with small bowel obstruction. It is not 'true faeces' that is vomited up (and it is often helpful to explain this to patients whose suffering is often compounded by disgust) but rather bowel contents altered by micro-oroganisms in the static bowel.

General points when taking the history

Is this the presenting symptom of cancer? Has the patient been referred to you by the general surgeons or medical team? If so, she will need an urgent explanation of her treatment options and detailed discussions in order to be able to manage her anxieties.

Conversely, has your patient had multiple courses of chemotherapy and is this the end of active life-prolonging treatments for her? Be careful to explain that you will actively treat her symptoms although you may no longer be able to take the disease away.

Key points on examination
General points

Is the patient in pain? Is it continuous or intermittent? Is the patient doubled up and/or holding her abdomen suggesting colicky pain?

- Is the patient mobile and active or bedbound, weak and exhausted?
- Is the patient cachectic?
- Is the patient dehydrated?

Abdominal examination

- Is the abdomen distended? Is this due to ascites or gaseous distension of the bowel?
- Is there generalized or focal abdominal tenderness? (Be gentle!)
- Are bowel sounds present? Are they normal?
- Check for abdominal guarding or rigidity.
- Is the rectum empty? If not, is it loaded with hard or very soft stool?
- Abdominal distention may be absent in high obstructions and when the bowel is 'plastered' down by extensive omental and mesenteric spread.

Investigations

Plain abdominal X-ray—this is often helpful in determining the site of intestinal obstruction or in differentiating a mechanical obstruction from an ileus and to look for faecal loading. An upright or lateral decubitus view of the abdomen should be included to look for air-fluid levels. A plain abdominal X-ray is also helpful to rule out constipation as a source of obstructive symptoms. *Plain films can underestimate the extent of disease progression; this is most accurately assessed by computerized tomography and/or bowel fluoroscopy.*

   X-rays may not be required if the patient is not being considered for surgery or if she is at the end of her life.

Management

Pain

The patient may be experiencing pain at the time of assessment. It is important that pain relief be provided without delay and throughout the balance of the patient's cancer experience. For moderate to severe abdominal pain, a strong opioid, such as morphine, administered on a regular basis, should be considered. It is likely that the patient will need parenteral opioids, which may be given by the subcutaneous or intravenous route. In Edmonton, the most usual regimen is intermittent bolus and in the UK, analgesia is given most commonly by continuous infusion. Subcutaneous administration is the preferred route. The dose of analgesic should be titrated on a regular basis until pain relief is achieved. Hyoscine butylbromide is effective for colicky abdominal pain: it can be used by bolus or constant infusion subcutaneously in a dose of 60–120 mg over 24 h. Breakthrough doses can be used within these parameters up to four times daily, if needed.

Table 7.1 Anti-emetic drugs (adapted from A. Spathis *Palliative Care Consultations in Haematology*, ch. 5. OUP.)

Drug	Indications	Mechanism of action	Dose	Comments
Metoclopramide	Functional bowel obstruction. Gastric stasis. Gastritis.	Prokinetic. D_2 antagonist + $5HT_4$ agonist. Prokinetic cholinergic nerves from myenteric plexus are inhibited by dopamine and stimulated by 5HT.	10 mg t.d.s. p.o. 30 mg/24 h CSCI	Effect blocked by antimuscarinic drugs e.g. cyclizine.
Haloperidol	Chemical causes of N + V including renal failure, drugs.	D_2 antagonist. Butyrophenone antipsychotic. Acts on chemoreceptor trigger zone, in area postrema, outside BBB.	1.5–2.5 mg o.d./b.d. p.o. 5 mg/24 h CSCI	Combines well with cyclizine. Useful in patients with anxiety, hallucinations, hiccups etc. Sedating.
Cyclizine	Mechanical bowel obstruction. Raised intracranial pressure. Movement related N + V.	Antihistaminic and antimuscarinic. Acts on vomiting centre, the central emetic pattern generator.	50 mg t.d.s. p.o. 150 mg/24 h CSCI	Can cause irritation at injection site. Can be sedating.
Hyoscine butylbromide	Mechanical bowel obstruction.	Antimuscarinic drug with both antispasmodic and antisecretory properties.	20 mg SC stat 60–120 mg/24 h CSCI Poorly absorbed p.o.	Not sedating as does not cross BBB. Useful in patients with bowel colic, excess respiratory secretions etc.

Levo-mepromazine	N + V of many causes.	Phenothiazine antipsychotic. Very broad spectrum: D_2, H_1, ACh, $5HT_2$ antagonist.	6–6.25 mg o.d./b.d, p.o./s.c. 6.25–25 mg/24 h CSCI Lasts 12–24 h (CSCI not necessarily needed)	'Nozinan' Usually substituted rather than added.
Dexamethasone	Multiple causes. Regurgitation due to oesophageal tumour, for example.	May reduce permeability of BBB to emetogenic substances. Anti-inflammatory effect.	4–8 mg o.d. p.o. or SC	Usually added to existing anti-emetic regimen.
Octreotide	Mechanical bowel obstruction.	Synthetic somatostatin analogue. Reduces bowel secretions and increases fluid absorption.	250–600 μg/24 h CSCI	Probably no more effective above 600 μg. Longer acting lanreotide now available (2 or 4 weekly injections).

N + V: nausea and vomiting. CSCI: continuous subcutaneous infusion. BBB: blood–brain barrier. RT: radiotherapy. o.d.: once daily. b.d.: twice a day. t.d.s.: three times a day. p.o.: by mouth. s.c.: subcutaneously.

Hydration

Artificial hydration is needed if the patient is suffering from dehydration or if surgery is being considered. Dehydration can cause or worsen delirium and trigger pre-renal failure, and this can result in opioid metabolite accumulation and toxicity.

Hypodermoclysis is an alternative to intravenous hydration, the latter is often difficult to establish and can be uncomfortable for patients with advanced cancer. Often only 1 l/day is required and the subcutaneous route can be easily established and maintained in the home.

Too much intravenous fluid can worsen symptoms and increase the volume of vomitus and intravenous hydration is not always needed.

Pharmacological Management

Pharmacotherapy is often extremely successful in palliating the symptoms associated with bowel obstruction in advanced gynaecological malignancy.

Nausea and vomiting

Nausea and vomiting may be controlled by either or both of two different pharmacological approaches:

- medications that reduce gastro-intestinal secretions, such as anticholinergics and/or somatostatin analogues; or
- anti-emetics alone or in association with medications to reduce gastro-intestinal secretions.

There are no comparative studies on the efficacy of these different approaches. Clinicians are often guided by their training, experience, drug availability and costs.

Anti-emetics (general)

Available anti-emetics for the management of malignant bowel obstruction include:

- prokinetic agents, e.g. metoclopramide and domperidone;
- neuroleptics—phenothiazines, butyrophenones (haloperidol);
- corticosteroids;
- anti-histaminic anti-emetics.

In some situations, a combination of anti-emetics with different sites of action can be used but it is counter-productive to use a prokinetic agent with an anti-histaminic agent, as the anti-emetic effects will be reduced.

Prokinetic agents

Metoclopramide This is an anti-dopaminergic prokinetic agent indicated in the management of bowel obstruction in the absence of abdominal colic—which it will worsen. It is particularly useful in dysmotility syndromes when it may reduce nausea and vomiting and aid in resolving the obstruction.

Metoclopramide is contra-indicated in bowel obstruction when the bowel lumen is occluded: to avoid this it should not be used when the patient has colic.

Methods of administration—Oral, subcutaneously (SC) or intravenously (IV) as intermittent bolus (Edmonton) or continuous infusion (more usual in the UK).

Possible side-effects include extrapyramidal effects such as rigidity and akasthisia but they are rare in clinical practice at normal therapeutic doses. Oculogryric crises are common in teenagers and the elderly.

Domperidone This is less likely to cause extrapyramidal side-effects than metoclopramide, as it does not cross the blood–brain barrier. As it is often only available in oral form, it may not be possible to use it in the setting of severe nausea or emesis.

Editor's note: In some countries, domperidone is available in a rectal formulation.

Neuroleptic agents

Phenothiazines The most important drug in this group for bowel obstruction is levomepromazine (methotrimeprazine). In some countries, low-dose methotrimeprazine is used as a first-line agent—but it is frequently used when other drugs have failed because of it tendency to cause drowsiness. Other possible phenothiazine side-effects include hypotension and Parkinsonism.

Chlorpromazine and prochlorperazine are too irritant to be given by subcutaneous infusion.

Levomepromazine is a long-acting drug and does not need to be given by continuous infusion—though it often is simply to avoid another injection. If it is the only drug needed it can be given once a day as a subcutaneous injection—a usual dose would be 6.25 mg to 12.5 mg—doses of 25 mg or more tend to cause troublesome sedation. There is a great inter-indiviudal variation in patient's tolerance of this.

Editor's note: This drug is not used in Edmonton for the management of bowel obstruction.

Butyrophenones Haloperidol is a potent suppressor of the chemoreceptor trigger zone. It has no direct effects on the gastro-intestinal tract and is commonly used as a first line agent in bowel obstruction. Haloperidol is less sedating and has fewer anticholinergic side-effects than the phenothiazines.

Corticosteroids

The role of corticosteroids in malignant bowel obstruction is complex and not well-defined. Besides possessing central anti-emetic effects, corticosteroids can also serve as co-analgesics and their anti-inflammatory effect may reduce peri-tumoural oedema and thereby increase the bowel lumen.

The most commonly used corticosteroid is dexamethasone because of its potency and limited mineralocorticoid effect. The dose range is 10–20 mg in divided doses per day IV/SC as boluses or by continuous SC infusion.

If a response is not seen in 4–5 days, the corticosteroid could be discontinued.

If a response is obtained, attempt to decrease the corticosteroid to the minimum effective dose to lessen the risk of side-effects, particularly as any response cannot, with certainty, be attributed to the steroid. A recent systematic review of the use of steroids in obstruction showed that '50% resolved on a placebo.'[7]

Antihistaminic agents

These include cyclizine, dimenhydrinate, diphenhydramine, and meclizine. In some countries, cyclizine is a first-line agent for the management of malignant bowel obstruction.

Potential side-effects of antihistaminic agents include sedation and anticholinergic effects.

Antisecretory agents (general)

Two classes of antisecretory agents with different mechanisms of actions are available:

(1) anticholinergics—hyoscine butylbromide, hyoscine hydrobromide (scopolamine), glycopyrrolate;

(2) somatostatin analogues—octreotide, vapreotide, lanreotide.

Anticholinergics

Hyoscine Butylbromide This drug is useful for the management of colicky abdominal pain. It decreases the tone of and peristalsis in smooth muscle.

It is also a potent antisecretory agent and reduces the volume of intestinal secretions. It can therefore help to reduce nausea and the frequency and volume of vomits especially in those with a proximal obstruction.

Methods of administration—SC or IV intermittently or by continuous infusion.

Side-effects—Hyoscine butylbromide is well tolerated. Central nervous system side-effects are few, as it is a quaternary ammonium compound and does not cross the blood-brain barrier easily.

Glycopyrrolate This can be substituted for hyoscine butylbromide. Glycopyrrolate is a more potent drying agent than hyoscine hydrobromide and also has few central nervous system side-effects because of its limited lipid solubility. It does not possess anti-emetic properties.[1–6]

Octreotide This is a somatostatin analogue that reduces gastro-intestinal secretions and bowel motility via the following mechanisms:

- reducing splanchnic blood flow;
- having a proabsorptive effect on water and ions;
- inhibiting the release of numerous hormones including gastrin, secretin, vasoactive intestinal peptide (VIP), and insulin.

The principal mechanism of fluid secretion in a bowel obstruction depends on VIP-induced inflammatory events. Octreotide has a potent anti-VIP effect.

Methods of administration—Octreotide can be given intermittently IV or SC (Edmonton). Continuous SC infusion is most usual in the UK.

Possible side-effects—These include local reactions at the site of injection, reduced glucose tolerance, and gastro-intestinal side-effects including nausea, vomiting, abdominal pain, bloating, diarrhea, steatorrhea, and anorexia. These side-effects are rarely clinically significant.

Octreotide may be effective in patients with a proximal bowel obstruction in whom hyoscine butylbromide has failed; it is often used in combination with hyoscine butylbromide. Research has shown that there is no advantage in using doses above 600 μm in 24 h.

Octreotide is expensive and is usually not considered first-line therapy except in patients with proximal obstruction. If a patient is being discharged to the community on these drugs it is wise (and polite) to contact the community physicians and nurses well before the patient goes home. Few will have much experience of its use in bowel obstruction.[8, 9]

Vapreotide This is a long-acting micro-encapsulated preparation of a somatostatin analogue with similar properties to octreotide. It has a longer duration of action and is administered weekly by intramuscular injection. It is available in only a few countries.

Lanreotide This is another somatostatin analogue with similar general properties to octreotide. It is given as a long-acting intramuscular depot injection and is primarily available in European countries. It may be used every 2–6 weeks depending on patient need.

> Long-acting somatostatin analogues should only be prescribed in patients with bowel obstruction after consultation with a specialist in palliative care

Why use a long-acting depot somatostatin analogue?

There is limited clinical experience available for these preparations but they probably have value for a number of individuals—especially those who are going to be discharged into the community.

In patients who will need octreotide for a prolonged period (weeks) it is often more economical and may be more convenient to use a depot preparation. If the patient is on multiple drugs in a syringe driver and a second driver may need to be started, then taking the somatostatin analogue out and using a depot preparation may remove the need for this. If the patient is only on octreotide (though this is rare) then the need for a driver may be removed completely.

General management

When the nausea, vomiting, and pain have been controlled by pharmacological therapy, the patient can often take fluids comfortably and may be put back on oral medication after a period of control on subcutaneous medication. No exact guidance can be given as to when the switch should be made but the patient's wishes are often the deciding factor. If she has had multiple episodes of bowel obstruction with repeated admissions, the patient will frequently prefer to stay on subcutaneous drugs rather than risk a resumption of symptoms she may well have come to dread. All patients need to be warned that recurrence of the symptoms is likely after one episode of obstruction and to ensure that they observe a palatable low residue diet, control constipation with laxatives, and report to their physician early for reassessment if they develop pain, or nausea and/or 'constipation'. There is little evidence for the effectiveness, or otherwise, of low-residue diets but a high-fibre diet is often felt, by clinicians, to add to the chances of re-obstruction. It is probably most important that the patient enjoys eating for her remaining lifespan and can have the social pleasure of small meals rather than concentrating on observing any sort of strict diet.

Subcutaneous infusions can be continued for weeks, even months at home. The infusion site should be changed at intervals—some drugs (such as levomepromazine) are more likely to cause skin irritation and the interval between site changes will be shorter.

Laxatives

Stimulant laxatives should be stopped in any patient with colic and faecal softeners should be used. Other conventional treatments for constipation such as purgatives and high enemas are contra-indicated. Constipation can only be treated in those patients with a known single rectal or colonic obstruction. These patients should be given a softening laxative.

Chemotherapy

The role of chemotherapy in ovarian cancer with intestinal obstruction is controversial. Many patients have been previously treated with chemotherapy, and the development of malignant bowel obstruction often represents progressive disease, with limited chemotherapeutic options.

Present thinking

Chemotherapeutic-naïve women with newly diagnosed ovarian cancer and inoperable malignant bowel obstruction are usually considered better candidates for chemotherapy.

Versus Chemotherapy is contra-indicated in gynaecological malignant bowel obstruction because of the poor performance status of many patients with this condition and problems that can occur with distribution of body fluids.[10]

Non-pharmacological management

Decompressive techniques

This should be considered for patients who have not responded to pharmacological management or to complement pharmacological management. The following techniques can be considered.

Nasogastric tube

A naso-gastric tube is often poorly tolerated and its use should be avoided where this is possible. If it is required, it should be used on a temporary basis to reduce secretions before the start of pharmacological treatment and during the first few days of such treatment. Long-term use should only be considered when drug therapy is ineffective and a venting gastrostomy, or other intervention, cannot be performed.

Complications associated with a nasogastric tube include nasal or pharyngeal irritation, aspiration pneumonia, oesophagitis, and gastritis or erosion, and bleeding.

Venting gastrostomy tube

This should be considered if medications are not successful in reducing vomiting. It is a more acceptable method for long-term decompression of an obstructed gastro-intestinal tract than a nasogastric tube and is used in a completely different way from a feeding gastrostomy.

Insertion This can be carried out during exploratory or palliative laparotomy, percutaneously by endoscopy, or using ultrasound or computed tomography guidance. It is rarely placed during surgery because medical treatment is usually successful, but it may be used where it becomes certain during surgery that obstruction will be permanent or where obstruction is inoperable and medical treatment has failed. Otherwise a percutaneous endoscopic gastrostomy (PEG) should be considered for the following reasons:

◆ there is a high success rate of insertion;

◆ it has a low morbidity and mortality;

◆ it is less costly;

◆ it avoids laparotomy.

The gastrostomy tube may allow the patient to drink clear fluids, although caution should be taken to avoid clogging. This, and dislodgement, is the commonest complication.

Relative contraindications to use These include the presence of massive carcinomatosis, portal hypertension and ascites, previous upper abdominal surgery, active gastric ulceration, and coagulopathy.

Potential complications are infrequent but can include hemorrhage, gastric perforation, gastrocolic fistula, stoma infections, and aspiration pneumonia.

Managing a venting gastrostomy

◆ The tube should be clamped during meals and for as long as this can be tolerated afterwards.

◆ Its output will fluctuate, presumably as the degree of obstruction changes.

◆ It can easily be managed at home, and patients have lived for months with a venting gastrostomy.[11]

Surgery

There is uncertainty regarding the benefits and possible harmful effects of surgery in patients with advanced disease and bowel obstruction. It should not be undertaken in all patients with advanced cancer and it will only benefit selected patients with mechanical obstruction. It is always an individual decision in which the patient's choice is paramount. The following must be considered:

◆ It is important to consider both whether palliative surgery is technically feasible and if the patient is likely to benefit from surgery.

◆ A single site of obstruction is uncommon in ovarian cancer. These patients are at risk of multiple levels of obstruction and where this is so, surgery is usually not feasible.

◆ A decision to operate should take into account the patient's wishes, anticipated survival, need for hospitalization, high morbidity and mortality of the procedure, and the potential failure to relieve obstruction.

Criteria for surgery and good prognostic variables include:

◆ a good performance status;

◆ no previous abdominal surgery other than resection of the primary tumor;

◆ recent onset of symptoms;

◆ low grade of tumor;

◆ long time-interval since the original operation;

◆ absence of ascites;

◆ younger age;

◆ a single site of occlusion;

◆ degree of secondary disease including previous radiotherapy and chemotherapy;

Absolute contra-indications to surgery include:

◆ a recent laparotomy demonstrating corrective surgery is not possible;

◆ re-obstruction;

◆ intra-abdominal carcinomatosis;

◆ poor nutritional status;

◆ poor general performance status;

◆ gross ascites that re-accumulates rapidly after paracentesis;

◆ if the patient does not want surgery that is only palliative in nature.

If surgery is chosen, the most appropriate approach depends on the level and cause of the obstruction. Single sites of obstruction are rare in gynaecological malignancy. When there is a single site of left-sided colonic obstruction, consider single-stage surgery: subtotal colectomy with primary anastomosis or partial colectomy with intra-operative lavage. If this treatment option is not possible, a two-stage procedure (Hartmann technique) may be performed. In advanced disease, a permanent colostomy should be considered.

Decompression of a severely distended colon may be achieved by a temporary colostomy. A complete mass or point of obstruction can be identified for complete tumor resection. A small bowel obstruction may be released or resected. In the presence of more extensive disease, the obstruction could be bypassed for palliation. Potential operative complications include the development of enterocutaneous fistulas, anastomotic leaks, short bowel syndrome, and sepsis.

In general, the decision to pursue surgical intervention should be made on an individual case basis. To help a patient make an informed decision, she should be provided with realistic information concerning expected effectiveness, likely and possible side-effects, and goals of treatment.[12, 13]

Metal stents

These are infrequently used in gynaecological malignancy as ovarian cancer is the most common cause and single sites of obstruction are rare in this condition. A colorectal stent should be considered for patients with a single colonic obstruction.

However, patients with widespread advanced cancer may not have clinical improvement after stent placement because of obstruction at other sites, multiple stenoses, or peritoneal carcinomatosis. Stent delivery—fluoroscopic screening for sigmoid and rectal tumors; proximal lesions may require a joint endoscopic and radiologic approach.

Well-conducted randomized trials are required to confirm efficacy, duration of effect, and possible cost saving advantages.[14, 15]

Parenteral nutrition

The considerations here are similar to those for surgical intervention—total parenteral nutrition (TPN) in the management of patients with inoperable bowel obstruction is controversial and should be used in selected patients only. The primary goal of TPN is to maintain or restore the patient's nutritional status and to correct or prevent malnutrition-related symptoms.

To date, it has not been proven that parenteral nutrition is beneficial in the care of patients with advanced cancer; protein anabolism is seldom achieved and weight gain is usually secondary to increases in body water and fat. However, there is a small subgroup of patients—young, affected by slow-growing tumors, with involvement of the gastro-intestinal tract, and sparing of the vital organs—who may die of starvation rather than tumor spread and for whom TPN may be considered.

The recommended variables for consideration of TPN include an estimated survival of >40 days and/or high-performance status at the beginning of treatment.

Potential TPN side-effects include promotion of bacterial translocation across the gastrointestinal tract, metabolic disturbances, and hepatic dysfunction.

Home TPN

This is labour intensive and expensive. It requires the active participation of the patient, the patient's family, nursing staff, and the patient's primary physician. Psychological support of the patient and her family is often required.[16, 17]

Conclusion

Pharmacological therapy is usually successful in palliating the symptoms of bowel obstruction in advanced gynaecological malignancy. Only highly selected patients with malignant bowel obstruction complicating a gynaecological cancer should be considered for surgery or parenteral nutritional supplementation. Obstruction is commonly found at multiple sites and dysmotility due to bowel wall or mesenteric obstruction and luminal obstruction frequently co-exist. Bowel obstruction is a relapsing and remitting condition and patients are often dead within six months of the first episode.

References

1 Ripamonti, C., Twycross, R., Baines, M., Bozetti, F., Capri, S. (2001). Clinical-practice recommendations for the management of bowel obstruction in patients with end-stage cancer. *Support Care Cancer*, **9**, 223–233.

2 Ripamonti, C. and Bruera, E. (2002). Palliative management of malignant bowel obstruction. *Int J Gynecol Cancer*, **12**, 135–143.

3 Rousseau, P. (1998). Management of malignant bowel obstruction in advanced cancer: a brief review. *J Palliative Medicine*, **1**, 65–72.

4 Mercadante, S. (1997). Assessment and management of mechanical bowel obstruction. In *Topics in palliative care*, vol.1 (Portenoy, R. K. and Bruera, E., ed.), pp. 113–130. Oxford University Press, New York.

5 Randall, T. C. and Rubin, S. C. (2000). Management of intestinal obstruction in the patient with ovarian carcinoma. *Oncology*, **14**, 1159–1163.

6 Ripamonti, C. (1994). Management of bowel obstruction in advanced cancer. *Curr Opinion Oncol*, **6**, 351–357.

7 Feuer, D. J. and Broadley, K. E. (2001). Corticosteroids for the resolution of malignant bowel obstruction in advanced gynaecological and gastrointestinal cancer. *The Cochrane Database of Systematic Reviews, The Cochrane Library, The Cochrane Collaboration*. Issue 2, pp. 1–27.

8 Ripamonti, C., Mercadante, S., Groff, L., Zecca, E., De Conno, F., and Casuccion, A. (2000). Role of octreotide, scopolamine, butylbromide, and hydration in symptom control of patients with inoperable bowel obstruction and nasogastric tubes: a prospective randomized trial. *J Pain Symptom Manage*, **19**, 23–34.

9 Ripamonti, C., Panzeri, C., Groff, L., Galeazzi, G., and Boffi, R. (2001). The role of somatostatin and ocreotide in bowel obstruction: pre-clinical and clinical results. *Tumori*, **87**, 1–9.

10 Abu-Rustum, N. R., Barakat, R. R., Venkatraman, E., and Spriggs, D. (1997). Chemotherapy and total parenteral nutrition for advanced ovarian cancer with bowel obstruction. *Gynecol Oncol*, **64**, 493–495.

11 Adelson, M. D. and Kasowitz, M. H. (1993). Percutaneous endoscopic drainage gastrostomy in the treatment of gastrointestinal obstruction from intraperitoneal malignancy. *Obstet Gynecol*, **81**, 467–471.

12 Feuer, D.J., Broadley, K. E., Shepherd, J. H., and Barton, D. P. J. (2001). Surgery for the resolution of symptoms in malignant bowel obstruction. *The Cochrane Database of Systematic Reviews, The Cochrane Library, The Cochrane Collaboration*. Issue 2, pp. 1–37.

13 Chen, L.-M. and Karlan, B. Y. (2000). Recurrent ovarian carcinoma: is there a place for surgery? *Semin Surg Oncol*, **19**, 62–68.

14 Ahmad, T. and Mee, A. S. (2000). Expandable metal stents in malignant colorectal obstruction. *BMJ*, **321**, 584–585.

15 Baron, T. H. (2001). Expandable metal stents for the treatment of cancerous obstruction of the gastrointestinal tract. *N Engl J Med*, **344**, 1681–1687.

16 Philip, J. and Depczynski, B. (1997). The role of total parenteral nutrition for patients with irreversible bowel obstruction secondary to gynecological malignancy. *J Pain Symptom Manage*, **13**, 104–111.

17 King, L. A., Carson, L. F., Konstantinidesm, N., Huuse, M. S., Adcock, L. L., Prem, K. A. *et al.* (1993). Outcome assessment of home parenteral nutrition in patients with gynecologic malignancies: what have we learned in a decade of experience? *Gynecol Oncol*, **51**, 377–382.

Chapter 8

Psychosexual problems in gynaecological malignancy

Lisa Punt

Introduction

The trauma of being given a diagnosis of a gynaecological malignancy and undergoing treatment for it can have an immense impact on a woman's psychosexual functioning. Feelings of uncertainty, depression, anxiety, and fear can be overwhelming, leaving her feeling completely isolated. These feelings may challenge a woman's concept of herself and threaten her social position, changing the balance of all her relationships. Her role as a mother, wife, carer, or partner may feel endangered, resulting in low self-esteem and a breakdown in communication, at a time when closeness and familiarity may offer sanctuary.

The disclosure of such feelings and concerns from our patients can often be inhibited by the nature of the clinical environment and the focus on physical treatment. Often healthcare professionals, at all levels, find time constraints, lack of privacy, and a lack of formal training deterrents to facilitating discussions surrounding the psychological impact of the disease and it's implications on normal functioning.

In 1947 the World Health Organization defined the word 'health' as being, 'not merely the absence of disease but a state of complete, physical, psychological and social well-being'.

We can often become overwhelmed with the desire to make the patient better, achieve a cure, or alleviate the physical symptoms without exploring the psychological changes that the woman may also be undergoing. This may result in an unhealthy patient, in spite of the disease being cured or physical symptoms adequately managed.

This chapter will explore some of the issues faced by women and their partners given such a diagnosis. It will also give guidance to all healthcare professionals who can influence the quality of life of women facing treatment for a gynaecological cancer.

Incidence of sexual dysfunction

Cancer survivorship among gynaecological oncology patients, in particular cervical and endometrial cancer, is relatively high. Around 45% of all cancer survivors have had a gynaecological malignancy.[2] This highlights that the long-term morbidity, which is likely to be both physical and psychological, needs to be addressed early in an attempt to limit its impact and allow women to gain the best possible quality of life following diagnosis and treatment.

Although scarce, research into the incidence of sexual dysfunction among gynaecological cancer patients shows a great variation. Some authors have found the incidence to be as high as 80%.[3] This demonstrates the enormous number of women, partners, and families who will be affected in some way by a change in sexual function following treatment for gynaecological cancer.

Normal sexual function

At this point it is timely to consider the definition of sexual dysfunction, since this allows us to consider that 'normal' will be an individual expectation, arising from one's own emotions, thought patterns, beliefs and values.

There are many different definitions of sexual dysfunction, but Clark in 1993 defined it as: 'The inability to express one's sexuality consistent with personal needs and preferences'.[4] This highlights the importance of establishing what the expectations of the patient and her partner are. For the healthcare professional it can sometimes be difficult to put aside their own beliefs and prejudices to ensure the needs of the individual are addressed.

For any individual her 'normal' sexual response will follow a specific pattern or cycle as described below. The length and intensity of each stage will be variable from one partnership to another.

- ◆ **Desire** is the primary sexual response cycle and can occur at different levels from uninterested through to active interest in sexual activities. Physical contact, visual stimuli and fantasising can all enhance the level of interest.

- ◆ **Excitement or arousal** is the second phase of the human response cycle. During this phase the woman's response to stimulation results in an increased blood flow to the genitals and an increase in vaginal lubrication. Parasympathetic nerve impulses then pass to the Bartholin glands, causing an increase in the mucous secretions at the introitus. The clitoris swells and enlarges, the vagina becomes longer and the uterus rises.

- ◆ **Orgasm** is the third phase, and peak of the cycle. Continued stimulation will result in this, the physical release of pleasurable expression.

During orgasm the muscles of the vagina, uterus, and sometimes the rectum, contract in a rhythmic pattern.

♦ Following orgasm there will be a *resolution* phase of relaxation where the capacity for arousal is inhibited.

For an individual to attain their 'normal' sexual function there must be an integration of three vital components: the nervous system, the vascular system, and the endocrine system.

If we consider the sexual response cycle to be analogous to that of an electrical circuit, then we are able to identify three primary potential breakpoints, any of which can lead to an interruption in the normal response cycle.

♦ The first breakpoint is **physical**. This can result from discomfort, pain, or inappropriate stimulation and will inhibit any possible further sexual response.

♦ The second breakpoint is **emotional**. This can occur when there is an over-whelming fear of failure, anxiety, anger, unresolved conflict, resentment, or guilt. This breakpoint can often be the most powerful and damaging.

♦ The third breakpoint is **mental**. Here the mind is intrusively preoccupied with negative experiences or worrying concerns. This will prevent the individual from relaxing and can also inhibit further sexual arousal.

The sexual response circuit may begin at any stage of the cycle, either physical, emotional, or mental but when any of these breakpoints are threatened then the normal sexual cycle can be disrupted and broken leading to sexual dysfunction.

Causes of sexual dysfunction following a diagnosis of cancer

There are many dimensions to cancer that can offer a threat to a woman's sexuality. The integration of psychological, behavioural, and physical changes are often difficult to separate and can make addressing sexual dysfunction a complex process.

Physical factors that will affect a woman who has undergone treatment may include damage resulting in functional changes, fatigue, and pain. Medications used to control pain, depression, or other treatment-related side-effects might also contribute to the direct physical effect of primary treatment.

The psychological impact may result from misunderstandings or misconceptions relating to the origin of the cancer (e.g. 'did I cause this cancer by having sex at an early age/many sexual partners?' or 'will I cause the cancer to come back by having sex?'), mood disturbances (e.g. fear, anxiety, or co-existing depression and changes in body image) can all offer a threat to the female sexual response.

Often presenting symptoms can be associated with sexual intercourse, e.g. post coital bleeding or dyspareunia (pain on intercourse). This can result in fear and preoccupation with disease association. What should be a pleasurable experience may now cause anxiety and fear of recurrence both for the patient and her partner.

Many patients with a gynaecological malignancy will undergo extensive treatment, and in the majority of cases multi-modality treatment. This may lead to a synergistic effect between the different treatment modalities and significantly increase the risk of physical damage to the pelvic and genital region.

Physical changes related to surgery

Hysterectomy ($+/-$ oophorectomy) will be the primary surgical treatment for a gynaecological malignancy. All pelvic surgery can affect sexual functioning by reducing the vascular supply to the pelvic organs, by removal of the pelvic organs, or by reducing the circulating hormones (see The menopause). Hysterectomy can sometimes result in a shortened vagina leading to dyspareunia associated with deep penile penetration. The sexual response cycle may also be broken due to the absence of rhythmic contractions of the uterus. This may inhibit or even prevent orgasm. Radical vulvectomy is a considerably more mutilating procedure, with the removal of the clitoris, labia, distal-third of the vagina, and possibly bilateral inguinal lymph node dissection. Such disfiguring surgery does not only have an immense impact on physical function but also on body image.

Physical changes related to chemotherapy

Many of the side-effects associated with chemotherapy can leave a women feeling asexual. These adverse effects include nausea, vomiting, constipation, diarrhoea, mucositis, fatigue, and alopecia (including the loss of pubic hair, which many women find distressing). Cytotoxic drugs have also been shown to reduce both vaginal lubrication and the ability to achieve orgasm. This is due, in part, to the induction of a premature menopause.

Physical changes related to radiotherapy

In the short term, radiotherapy can result in side-effects such as fatigue, nausea, vomiting, diarrhoea, and perineal soreness, all of which may contribute to a loss of desire during a course of radiotherapy treatment.

Radiotherapy can also cause chronic side-effects that can continue to affect a woman for many years following her initial treatment. Direct damage to the vaginal mucosa, both from external beam and/or brachytherapy can result in a thinning of the basal cell layer within the vagina. Vaginal stenosis results from the formation of adhesions and fibrosis of the vaginal tissue. These changes will lead to shortening and narrowing of the vaginal vault.

For women undergoing radiotherapy to the vagina it is essential that information and education be offered on reducing the risk of vaginal stenosis. Vaginal dilation will minimize the formation of adhesions and help to minimize the build-up of scar tissue. This can be achieved either with the regular use of vaginal dilators or/and sexual intercourse.

Telangiectasia can also occur, particularly in the upper-third of the vagina, leading to contact bleeding—a symptom that may have led the women to seek medical attention prior to diagnosis. Irradiating the ovaries will result in a woman entering the menopause, which will also have a direct effect on sexual function (see under menopause)

The menopause

Many women undergoing treatment for a gynaecological malignancy will be faced with a treatment-induced, or early menopause. The implications of this can be far-reaching for a women who is not only dealing with a life-threatening disease, but also facing a process associated with growing old and the issues surrounding the loss of fertility.

Many women who are peri- or post-menopausal will note a change in sexual desire. The effect that changing oestrogen and androgen levels have on sexual desire is poorly understood, however they clearly have a role to play. Following oophorectomy, the circulating serum androgen levels are shown to be reduced by up to 34%. Current thinking is that there is a synergistic effect between androgens and oestrogen to promote libido.[5]

Circulating oestrogen also plays an important role in the maintenance of the healthy vaginal mucosa. Declining levels of oestrogen will result in senile changes that include shortening and narrowing of the vaginal vault, reduced vaginal blood flow, loss of lubrication, increased pH due to loss of glycogen, and atrophy of the vaginal vault.

These atrophic changes resulting from a lack of oestrogen can lead to dyspareunia which, if left untreated, will affect the physical primary break-point of the sexual response cycle, leading to sexual dysfunction or a reduction in the frequency of intercourse.

Oral hormone replacement therapy can be offered to those women who are being treated for an oestrogen-receptor negative tumour. If vaginal atrophy continues, or there is persistent vaginal irritation or infection, then it may be necessary to offer topical oestrogen cream to be used directly on the vaginal mucosa. This is often required if the blood supply to the vagina has been compromised by surgery and/ or radiotherapy.

Addressing sexual dysfunction

Sexual health is the integration of the somatic, emotional, intellectual and social aspects of sexual beings in ways that are positively enriching and enhance personality, communication and love.

The World Health Organization (1975).[6]

We, as healthcare professionals, are in a privileged position. We are afforded the opportunity to influence positively the rehabilitation of women undergoing treatment for a gynaecological malignancy.

Many women will find it difficult to discuss concerns about sexuality when they attend for hospital visits. Likewise, many medical staff, radiographers, and nurses may feel uneasy or lack the skills to facilitate a discussion surrounding sexual function and psychological adjustment.

An inability on our part to show acceptance for discussing sexual health at this point will only confirm to the patient that such issues are a taboo subject and that her concerns should not be raised in the clinical environment. This fear of unacceptability may result in a lack of basic information being provided for the patient at an early stage.

For example, when women are encouraged to resume intercourse soon after completing treatment, they will often express concern that they may cause the cancer to come back or contaminate their partner with either the cancer or the radiation, or even cause damage following a surgical procedure. These misunderstandings, if uncorrected with accurate information, will lead on to a change in sexual function purely due to a lack of understanding of the disease and its treatment.

The difficulties that healthcare professionals face when dealing with sexuality can be diverse and far-reaching. Few of us are 'taught', or have the experience in dealing with, such issues during our professional education. Very few post-graduate courses are available and the research and literature is scarce. It is no wonder that our own inadequacies can lead us to feel anxious and reticent about approaching a subject with which we may feel uncomfortably out of our depth.

Apart from training issues, time and space can also be limiting factors in a busy clinical department.

Just as normal sexual function relies on a complex interplay of physical and emotional well-being, addressing sexual dysfunction carries with it a responsibility to provide an holistic approach.

A sensitive and informed approach to facilitating discussions surrounding sexuality can provide effective support to women and their partners before, during, and after treatment for a gynaecological malignancy. An empathetic relationship between the patient and her healthcare professional is essential to encompass the vast intergrational needs of the individual.

Carl Roger defines empathy as, 'the ability to experience another person's world as if it were one's own, without losing the "as if".'

When used effectively, an empathetic response can provide an environment in which the patient/couple feel safe and comfortable discussing issues surrounding sexual function and any concerns they may have following treatment. An ability to understand another's needs and expectations is a skill that will allow a timely delivery of appropriate information at a level that is understood by the woman and her partner.

A framework of varying levels of complexity that can be employed to help healthcare professionals provide sexual assessment and rehabilitation is the PLISSIT model.[7] This is best shown as a diagrammatic pyramid (Fig. 8.1). The area of each level indicates the proportion of healthcare professionals who should be able to provide that level of intervention.

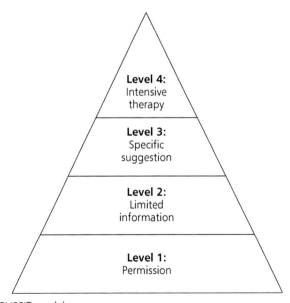

Fig. 8.1 The PLISSIT model.

Level 1: Permission giving

At this level all healthcare professionals should recognize that sexual issues are an integral part of a person's well-being and, are therefore acceptable to acknowledge and discuss with those facing a life-threatening disease.

Even if the medical professional and/or patient may not wish to discuss intimate details, the patient can be given the opportunity to raise concerns by using 'matter of fact' general statements relevant to possible sexual dysfunction following their diagnosis and treatment.

The examples set out below are designed to summarize the factual information that may be given at 'permission giving' level, they are not intended to be examples of the way in which the information should be given. The reader should employ all their communication skills and hone these as needed. For example:

> During your operation it will be necessary to remove your ovaries. This will result in you experiencing an early menopause. As a result of your declining oestrogen levels some women find that they have a decrease in sexual desire.

> After your radiotherapy is complete, there may be changes to the vagina that can result in a build up of scar tissue. For some woman this can result in sexual intercourse feeling different.

Both of the above statements contain information that is necessary for informed consent prior to treatment. However, it is the manner in which the information is delivered that will determine the success of facilitating a timely discussion with the woman.

When important information about the impact of treatment is given, such as in the above examples, it may not be appropriate for a woman to discuss issues surrounding sexuality at such an early stage in her diagnosis. Also, the clinician consenting the patient may not be the most appropriate person to discuss further concerns. However, we must all take responsibility for giving permission for a woman to discuss a subject with which many of us feel uncomfortable.

One approach may be to identify and acknowledge the potential issues and allow the woman to take some control over the timing of further discussions. For example:

> We are aware that the side-effects we have mentioned may cause some difficulties for you and your partner, and it is important that we give you information on how you can minimize some of these changes. This is something we can talk about now or later in your treatment, how do you feel about this?

Not only is this showing acceptance of the subject, but also a willingness to discuss it and for the patient to have some control over when this happens.

Level 2: Limited information

At this level the patient can be encouraged to explore the potential side-effects resulting from their treatment. The medical professional may give information about the changes that are likely to take place and offer education on proposed solutions. For example:

- By giving a clear explanation about the effects of oestrogen loss on the vaginal mucosa, it is possible for a woman and her partner to understand why there may be a lack of sensation during intercourse, or why the vagina remains dry even during the excitement phase of intercourse. This apparent lack of 'response' to stimulation can often leave a partner feeling inadequate and a woman feeling uncertain of why her physical response is different.

- The use of topical oestrogen cream and/or lubricating jelly can help to improve lubrication and, together with an understanding of the reasons behind the changes, help to prevent a break in the sexual response cycle.

Level 3: Specific suggestion

Using this level of intervention, the medical professional should be able to respond to any specific concerns raised by the woman and/or her partner. Suggestions on minimizing the effects of treatment should be given. For example:

It is possible to reduce the build up of scar tissue within the vagina, and this will help to minimise discomfort during intercourse. By using vaginal dilators you will prevent the walls of the vagina adhering to one another. For a while after treatment, you may still find intercourse uncomfortable and it may be necessary to try a different position during intercourse to allow you to control the depth of penetration and minimize the pressure on the cervix or the top of the vagina.

Level 4: Intensive therapy

A woman (or couple) who has a history of pre-existing concerns surrounding sexuality often requires a more intense level of intervention. There may be a history of abuse or sexual difficulties within their relationship prior to a diagnosis of cancer. Referral for psychological or sexual therapy is often appropriate, as long-term counselling will commonly be indicated.

When dealing with sexual health issues it is of fundamental importance that there are adequate routes of referral available for those individuals or couples who require more intense and prolonged therapy.

It is also essential that, whilst aiming to establish best practice and provide a high level of service, we also remain aware of our own individual limitations and inhibitions, in order not to influence or prejudice the health of the patient.

Conclusion

As we strive continually to improve and further develop a multidisciplinary team approach to cancer care, we need to embrace the skills of all team members. The holistic approach needed to address sexual dysfunction will be best managed in a supportive, multi-professional group, where referral to a psychosexual counsellor is available.

More then ever before we are aware of the need to care for the patient as a whole, addressing not just the physical well-being, but also the spiritual and emotional needs of the individual. Yet many barriers still exist within the clinical setting that inhibit good psychosexual care.

If we can identify those areas that hinder and prevent psychosexual support, such as time, space, and staff training, then we are in a stronger position to break down the barriers. Only then can we begin to provide a truly 'holistic' approach to cancer care.

References

1. Maughan, K. and Clarke, C. (2001). The effect of a clinical nurse specialist in gynaecological oncology on quality of life and sexuality. *Journal of Clinical Nursing*, **10**(2), 221–229.

2 Anderson, B. L. (1996). Predicting and treating sexual difficulties of gynaecological cancer survivors. *Cancer Control*, **3**(2), 113–119.

3 Anderson, B. L. and van Der Does, J. (1994). Surviving gynaecological cancer and coping with sexual morbidity: an international problem. *Int J Gynaecol Cancer*, **4**, 225–240.

4 Clark, J. C. (1993). Psychosocial responses of the patient: altered sexual health. In *Cancer nursing principles and practice*, 3rd edition (S. I. Groenwald, M. H. Frogge, and M. Goodway), pp. 449–467. Boston: Jones and Bartlett.

5 Nachtigall, L. (1994). Treatment of the postmenopausal woman: basic and clinical aspects. *Sexual function in the menopause and postmenopause*, pp. 301–306. Rogerio A. Lobo. Raven Press Ltd.

6 Rice, A. (2000). Sexuality in cancer and palliative care 2: exploring the issues. *Int J of Palliative Care*, **6**: 448–453.

7 Annon, J. S. (1976). *Behavioral treatment of sexual problems: brief therapy*. Hagerstown, Maryland: Harper & Row.

Chapter 9

Thrombosis and bleeding problems in gynaecological malignancy

Dawn L. Alison

Summary

Venous thrombo-embolism (VTE) and bleeding problems are important causes of morbidity and mortality in patients with cancer. Both give rise to distressing symptoms and their management in patients with advanced disease can be difficult.

Patients can experience clotting and bleeding problems at the same time and gynaecological cancer patients are at particular risk of this because of the sites of their cancers and patterns of metastatic spread. Providing the best care for such patients requires careful consideration of the individual patient's circumstances—her views must always be taken into account when planning management.

There is a wealth of published papers reporting the incidence, investigation, and treatment of VTE and bleeding in cancer patients undergoing active anticancer treatment but relatively little about the same issues in patients with advanced disease.

Thrombosis in advanced gynaecological malignancy

Thrombosis

It has long been recognized that cancer is associated with thrombo-embolic syndromes.[1] There is increasing knowledge of the contributing causes, which include changes in the factors involved in the complex thrombogenesis cascade. Platelet activation by tumour cells leading to adhesion or aggregation, procoagulant generation by tumour cells and inflammatory cells, increased levels of clotting factors I, V, VII, IX, and XI, and possible reduction of inhibitors such as antithrombin III, protein C, and protein S may all play their part in disturbing the balance of coagulation and fibrinolysis.

Patients with the most common gynaecological cancers (ovarian, uterine corpus, and uterine cervix) frequently have other major risk factors for the development of thrombo-embolism. In advanced disease these include:

- pelvic masses compressing large veins;
- reduced mobility (associated with surgery, ascites and leg lymphoedema secondary to pelvic lymph node metastases or radiotherapy);
- treatments such as surgery, radiotherapy, and chemotherapy (sometimes including the additional risk of an indwelling central venous cannula);
- occasionally hormone therapy (in particular tamoxifen, which may be used as a second- or third-line treatment in ovarian cancer).

The frequency with which venous thrombo-embolic complications arise in patients with gynaecological cancers is not known precisely but is probably underestimated. In one reported series, deep vein thrombosis (DVT) occurred in up to 45% patients after surgery for advanced ovarian and vulvar cancers.[2] In another series, 10.6% of patients with ovarian cancer undergoing chemotherapy developed a DVT[3] and post-mortem studies have described pulmonary emboli (PE) in 34.6% of ovarian cancer patients. In the general population it is reported that approximately 40% of patients with DVT have a pulmonary embolism.

Rarely patients may experience arterial thrombo-embolic problems.

Assessment of thrombotic problems

Individual signs and symptoms are of little use in the diagnosis of DVT but patterns of signs and symptoms can be useful. Clinical scoring systems have been devised taking account of these to help guide diagnosis and subsequent investigation. An example of this is the clinical rule devised by Wells and colleagues in which points are added or deducted for certain risk factors.[4] A point is added for each of the following:

- active cancer (continuing treatment or treatment completed within previous 6 months or palliative care patient);
- paralysis, paresis, or recent plaster immobilization of the lower extremities;
- recently bedridden for more than 3 days or major surgery within 4 weeks;
- localized tenderness along the distribution of the deep venous system;
- swelling of the entire leg;
- calf swollen by more than 3 cm when compared with the asymptomatic leg (measured 10 cm below the tibial tuberosity);
- pitting oedema (greater in the symptomatic leg);
- collateral superficial veins (non-varicose).

Two points are deducted if an alternative diagnosis is as likely or greater than that of deep vein thrombosis.

- If 0 points are scored, the risk category is low with a 3% probability of DVT (95% confidence intervals 2–6%).

- If 1–2 points are scored, the risk category is moderate with a 17% probability of DVT (95% confidence intervals 12–23%).

- If the score is greater than 2, the risk category is high with a 75% probability of DVT (95% confidence intervals 63–84%).

Important points in history

Careful assessment of gynaecological cancer patients with suspected venous thrombosis is needed as limb swelling or symptoms suggestive of thromboembolic complications (such as pulmonary emboli) may be caused by other malignancy-related problems or unrelated illnesses. Lymphoedema or dependent oedema in patients with co-existing cardiovascular disease can make diagnosis difficult, as can oedema due to reduced mobility and hypoproteinaemia. A high index of suspicion is needed, and known predisposing risk factors should be sought, in the history; for example, recent surgery, chemotherapy, radiotherapy, or hormonal therapy. Checking for previous episodes of venous thrombosis should be included. Features that may suggest development of DVT include a rapid onset of swelling and new pain or discomfort in a limb.

Clinical patterns of PE include sudden collapse or faintness, pleuritic pain, and/or haemoptysis or isolated dyspnoea. Specific enquiry about these should be made, remembering that PE is easily missed—particularly in the presence of severe cardiorespiratory disease, in elderly patients, and when the only symptom is breathlessness.

Patients should also be asked about previous illnesses that may affect the management of thrombo-embolic disease; for example, previous or current peptic ulcer disease—particularly if it has been complicated by bleeding.

A detailed medication history will reveal the potential for drug interactions and any contra-indications for oral anticoagulant therapy. Taking such a history will also highlight those patients who have needed complex symptom control regimens and where symptom control has been hard won. This is important as it may influence the decision on whether or not oral anticoagulation should be initiated. Attaining therapeutic levels for this treatment can sometimes be difficult, requiring frequent venous sampling and changes of anticoagulant dose. This can have a detrimental effect on a patient's quality of life.

Important points on examination

A careful physical examination is always necessary, although it is impossible to exclude the presence of DVT by clinical examination alone. There is no diagnostic sign for DVT—Homan's sign has long been discredited.

The patient's general condition should be assessed with particular attention to her nutritional state, level of discomfort, mobility, and cognitive function, as these will be important considerations when deciding appropriate investigations and possible treatment strategies.

Clothing and hosiery should be removed to allow full exposure of the limbs to be examined. An assessment of the extent of limb swelling, skin colour and temperature, and the presence of dilated superficial veins and lymphadenopathy should be recorded.

Venous thrombosis is more likely if the limb appears dusky, feels warm, has superficially dilated veins, and has become swollen and tender recently. By contrast, lymphoedema will cause more gradual swelling and the limb will not be warm or painful unless cellulitis has developed.

Bilateral lower limb swelling may signify lymphatic obstruction in the retroperitoneum caused by tumour masses or nodal disease. Inferior vena cava compression may cause a similar appearance and it can be difficult to determine if thrombosis has developed.

The abdomen should be inspected for the presence of distended veins, swelling of the abdomen, vulva and perineum, and abdominal wall oedema.

Vaginal examination This may provide information that will help both with making a diagnosis and deciding future management. This examination will enable the clinician to assess tumour masses in the pelvis, the vaginal vault, and/or in the vaginal wall For example, the presence of a friable tumour mass in the vagina, which bleeds on contact, may alter the risk/benefit ratio for an individual patient when anticoagulation is being considered.

Examination of the cardiovascular and respiratory systems is essential to detect and assess co-morbid conditions. In particular, clinicians should look for tachypnoea, pleural effusions, consolidation, raised jugular venous pressure, and other signs of right-sided heart failure, which could be caused by pulmonary emboli.

Possible investigations

Before subjecting a patient to any investigations it is essential to know that the results will influence treatment for that individual or contribute to planning her overall care by, for example, providing prognostic information. This is particularly important in palliative care practice. If the results will not alter these then the investigations should not be done.

The patient's goals are central to her management and careful discussion should take place to learn her views on investigations and possible treatments before any further steps are taken. The patient should be offered information about the doctor's clinical assessment, and the options for treatment and symptom management including the risks and perceived benefits. The balance of risks versus possible benefits will be different for each woman. Even investigations that do not seem invasive to a doctor may not be considered worthwhile by a patient.

For example, a woman with very advanced disease, who has an estimated prognosis of days to weeks, and who is being cared for at home and spending most of her time in bed may not wish to undergo the journey to hospital for radiological investigation For her, the possible benefits of anticoagulation may not be outweighed by the burdens of additional blood tests or daily injections that anticoagulation would necessitate if the diagnosis of DVT is confirmed. It would be sensible to know the patient's view about this at the outset.

The gold standard for diagnosis of DVT is contrast venography but this has been replaced generally by use of Doppler ultrasound. This has the attraction of being a non-invasive technique, but it is less accurate for distal DVTs that are of less clinical importance. Magnetic resonance scanning can also be used. Local resources and expertise will dictate the choice of investigation.

Whole-blood D-dimer estimation is also useful in the diagnosis of DVT. D-dimers are degradation products of cross-linked fibrin, and levels are elevated in DVT. The sensitivity of the test is 90–95% but the specificity only 55%. Therefore the test is best suited to ruling out DVT rather than proving its presence. It is also recommended that D-dimer estimation is used as an adjunct to other diagnostic methods because when used alone the test will fail to diagnose 5–10% DVTs.

D-dimer levels are often elevated in cancer patients and so its usefulness in the investigation of suspected DVT in this group has been questioned. A recent study investigating the clinical utility of whole-blood rapid D-dimer tests in cancer patients with suspected DVT compared with non-cancer patients concluded that the negative predictive value seemed as high in the cancer patients as in the non-cancer ones.[5]

A possible diagnostic strategy in a patient with advanced gynaecological cancer suspected of having DVT would include D-dimer estimation with compression ultrasonography. If both tests are normal, a DVT is not likely. If the D-dimer test result is abnormal, repeat the ultrasonogram a week later. If this test is normal, a DVT can again be ruled out.

Computed tomographic (CT) scans with contrast will also demonstrate thromboses and sometimes a scan undertaken for disease staging, or to assess response to therapy, will reveal a thrombosis that is not apparent clinically. This is most often the case when lower limb swelling has been present for some time due to other cancer-related effects such as lymphadenopathy or venous compression from tumour masses in the pelvis. In such circumstances it can be difficult to detect the effects of insidious occlusive thrombus formation.

Suspected PE If a PE is suspected, investigations and interim therapy awaiting a firm diagnosis will depend on the clinical picture as previously discussed. The presence of advanced cancer is both a major risk factor for the development of PE and an important reason to modify standard management algorithms.

Definitive investigations for PE include pulmonary angiography, ventilation perfusion lung scans (if plain chest radiograph is normal), and pulmonary spiral CT scanning (helpful in the presence of abnormal plain chest radiogram). All of these investigations are available only in the hospital setting; for patients who are either at home or are being cared for in a hospice, the decision to undertake specialist investigation will require careful thought and discussion. The same consideration should be given to decisions about hospital in-patients, as the ease with which clinicians can arrange an investigation should not be the major factor in deciding if it is done.

Other useful investigations in patients with suspected DVT or PE include a full blood count, electrocardiogram, plain chest radiograph, serum albumin levels, and tests of liver function and clotting. These may provide evidence that supports the diagnosis of pulmonary embolism or may point towards other possible explanations for the symptoms. Knowing the results of clotting tests and liver function tests will guide decisions about which method of anticoagulation is used (and drug doses) if a DVT or PE is confirmed.

Assessment—who else can help?

The need to have the patient's view about the extent to which she is prepared to undergo investigation or treatment has already been emphasized. Her decision may, in turn, be influenced by whether or not further palliative anticancer treatment is available. This information can be sought from clinical or medical oncology colleagues.

Management of thrombosis

Dealing with diagnostic uncertainty is difficult and, as previously described, making the diagnosis of venous thrombo-embolism in patients with advanced cancer is complicated. It requires an individual approach for each patient and, because definitive investigations cannot always be done, clinical assessment may be the only basis on which a diagnosis can be made. When the therapies are potentially burdensome and toxic, but the risk of non-treatment may also contribute to increased morbidity and mortality, the clinical decision-making is challenging and requires skilled communication. The complexities have been well described in a review of practice of palliative physicians.[6] Issues to be considered were summarized as:

◆ the appropriateness of anticoagulation;

◆ the most appropriate anticoagulant;

◆ the duration of anticoagulation.

Drug therapy

Treatment for venous thrombo-embolism is aimed at preventing:

◆ local extension of thrombus;

◆ embolization (with its high risk of fatality);

◆ recurrent thrombosis.

The drug treatments available are:

◆ anticoagulant therapy, which can prevent growth of an existing thrombus or embolus; or

◆ thrombolytic therapy to accelerate dissolution of thrombi or emboli.

Anticoagulants The optimal method of anticoagulation for DVT in patients with advanced gynaecological cancer is not known. The standard approach involves initial treatment with an intravenous infusion (or three times daily subcutaneous injections) of full-dose unfractionated heparin or a once daily subcutaneous injection of low molecular weight heparin (e.g. tinzaparin). This treatment is usually prescribed for 5–7 days and oral anticoagulation with warfarin is commenced after 24–48 h. An overlap of treatments is recommended to ensure that the international normalized ratio (INR) of prothrombin time (used for monitoring warfarin dose) has been within the therapeutic range for 2 consecutive days. Warfarin therapy may then be continued for a variable time in order to prevent recurrent venous thrombo-embolism.

In patients with advanced cancer this approach may not be the most suitable for reasons summarized below.

Unfractionated heparin. Use of unfractionated heparin has several potential disadvantages. First it requires daily monitoring with blood sampling to check the activated prothrombin time (APTT) with the aim of keeping this in the range 1.5–2.5 of the control level. Some patients will find this burdensome and uncomfortable, particularly if venous access is difficult. Similarly, the intravenous administration or subcutaneous injections three times daily may be inconvenient.

Second, unfractionated heparin can cause thrombocytopenia, increasing the risk of haemorrhage associated with any anticoagulant treatment. Finally, it can also cause osteoporosis after prolonged use. This may occasionally be of significance for patients treated with heparin on several occasions within a few months or for a longer time than is usual because they have developed recurrent thrombo-embolism, despite oral anticoagulation.

Low molecular weight heparin (LMWH). This is an easier treatment than warfarin, as a weight-adjusted dose gives a predictable anticoagulant effect so that repeated blood sampling is not needed. The exception to this is in very obese patients or patients with severe renal dysfunction.

LMWH has other advantages. Its main anticoagulant effect is as an anti-factor X agent. Additionally, its higher bioavailability and longer half-life than unfractionated heparin after subcutaneous injection allows for once or twice daily injection, depending on the preparation. Low molecular weight heparins are excreted mainly by the kidneys and are less likely to cause thrombocytopenia and osteoporosis. They are however more expensive.

Warfarin. This is a 4-hydroxycoumarin compound and is the oral anticoagulant most commonly used for prolonged anticoagulation. However, its use in patients with advanced cancer has been questioned.[7] It inhibits the synthesis of factors dependent on vitamin K (prothrombin or factor II, factors VII, IX, X, protein C, and protein S). It is 97% bound to albumin and its metabolism takes place in the liver, a water-soluble inactive metabolite being excreted in bile. These properties contribute to the difficulties of using warfarin in cancer patients in whom hepatic function and nutritional status may be reduced. Its variability of effect is influenced by age, racial background, diet, and use of many other drugs. Frequent monitoring with repeated venepunctures is thus a necessity but potentially intrusive for terminally ill patients.

Warfarin therapy is monitored by assessing the ratio of a patient's prothrombin time to a standard. This is the international normalized ratio (INR). Although different levels of INR have been recommended for different clinical situations, a recent review of this practice supports a uniform approach aiming for an INR close to 2.2–2.3 because of the observed excess mortality associated with high INR values.[8] Difficulties maintaining a target INR in palliative care practice are common.[6]

Thrombolytic therapy Thrombolytic therapy uses drugs to lyse thrombus, either by potentiating the body's own thrombolytic pathways or by mimicking natural thrombolytic pathways. Streptokinase and recombinant plasminogen activator are examples of these agents. Their lack of specificity and associated risk of haemorrhage means they are unlikely to be indicated in patients with advanced gynaecological cancer. Most patients will have one or more absolute or relative contra-indications such as recent or current haemorrhage, coagulation defects, liver disease, or heavy vaginal bleeding.

Thrombolytic therapy may be appropriate for that small group of patients who develop arterial thrombosis. In these women, arterial catheterization and targeted drug delivery can resolve thrombus sufficiently to provide satisfactory distal perfusion and prevent the distress of distal limb gangrene or amputation.[9]

Other medical therapy

Effective analgesia is an essential goal of management for every patient. Simple analgesics, such as paracetamol, may be enough for some with the addition of weak opioids if this is ineffective (e.g. codeine at optimal doses). Strong opioids, such as morphine, fentanyl, or oxycodone should be introduced and titrated to effect for patients whose pain is still poorly controlled. Non-steroidal anti-inflammatory drugs (NSAIDs) may be useful as co-analgesics but they are generally contra-indicated in patients taking anticoagulants because of the increased risk of haemorrhage.

Vena caval filters The placement of a vena caval filter in cancer patients with venous thrombo-embolism (especially if it is recurrent) is favoured by some clinicians. In particular, their use is recommended for patients who have a high risk for PE but who also have a high risk of a substantial bleed (or who are actively bleeding), so that anticoagulation can be avoided. Patients presenting with a deep vein thrombosis at the time of their diagnosis with advanced gynaecological cancer may also benefit from pre-operative placement of a filter if it is feasible. In patients with poor prognosis, advanced progressive disease the discomfort, risk, and expense of filter placement may not be associated with any significant gains.

Important palliative care points

Distal DVTs carry a low risk of embolization. Symptomatic management is a reasonable approach in patients with advanced cancer, although it should be borne in mind that extension of the clot to more proximal veins may occur.

The patient should be advised to elevate her swollen limb when at rest, as this will help to relieve the symptoms.

It is also important to pay attention to skin care to avoid further complications, and patients should be advised to try to avoid skin damage (e.g. when cutting their nails, gardening, etc.) and to use bland non-perfumed moisturizing creams, and to treat skin infections promptly.

Compression garments, sometimes used to manage lymphoedema, and deep massage should be avoided, although lightweight support hosiery and superficial light massage are unlikely to cause problems.

The choice of treatment for gynaecological cancer patients with venous thrombo-embolism will depend on the individual circumstances. Earlier discussion has outlined the difficulties associated with warfarin. An additional consideration is that warfarin may not be the most effective anticoagulant in cancer patients, as re-thrombosis rates have been noted to be as high as 16% in cancer patients, despite warfarin therapy. This fits with the experience described by many clinicians that patients with cancer and venous thrombo-embolism need a higher INR than patients with non-malignant disease to prevent recurrence.

The mechanism for the development of venous thrombo-embolism in cancer patients is probably chronic low-grade disseminated intravascular coagulation (DIC) leading to a compensatory increase in clotting factors. Heparin may be more effective as an anticoagulant in such cases.

Patients with advanced gynaecological cancers may also have other symptoms that are difficult to manage and this will influence choice of treatment. Pelvic pain, inadequately managed by other methods, may benefit from interventional pain control procedures such as spinal analgesia or peripheral nerve blocks. Patients with recurrent ascites may need repeated abdominal paracenteses. In all these situations, quick reversal of anticoagulant drug effects is desirable and the use of low molecular weight heparin has clear advantages over warfarin here. Omitting the daily dose of LMWH and waiting 24 h are usually all that is required, whereas normalization of the INR can take several days after stopping warfarin unless agents to reverse its effects are given.

Travel Patients with advanced cancer quite commonly wish to take a final holiday abroad with their family or friends. There are two factors to consider in such cases. Air travel and prolonged immobility on coaches or trains will add to a patient's risk for developing venous thrombo-embolism, so prophylactic anticoagulation may be sensible. For patients already anticoagulated because of previous DVT it is likely to be easier to manage anticoagulation safely using LMWH than using warfarin, as arranging monitoring of treatment whilst away may be possible but may prove difficult to organize.

The guidelines for the duration of anticoagulant treatment for patients with venous thrombo-embolism in the general population do not apply for patients with advanced cancer where the risks of VTE will continue and probably increase with disease progression. Decisions about stopping treatment will probably be most influenced by a patient's general deterioration and a desire to simplify medication and interventions as death approaches. Also, complications of treatment such as haemorrhage (even if fairly minor) may lead to a patient wishing to stop treatment, as even small bleeding episodes can be alarming for a patient coping with other unpleasant and frightening symptoms.

The evidence available on the treatment of venous thrombo-embolism in patients with advanced cancer suggests that the use of low molecular weight heparin is the treatment of choice for most patients.

Bleeding problems in patients with advanced malignancy

There are many reasons why patients with gynaecological cancer may suffer from bleeding problems.

1   **Advanced disease.** Bleeding occurs commonly as a presenting symptom of gynaecological cancer, particularly in patients with uterine body and cervical cancers. In countries where screening programmes for cervical cancer are poorly developed or non-existent, patients may present with advanced disease and massive haemorrhage may occur. Relapsed disease can also cause troublesome vaginal bleeding and, in patients with ovarian cancer, it can signal the development of vaginal vault metastases. Spread of uterine and cervical cancers may also lead to bladder or lower bowel invasion sometimes with associated bleeding problems.

2   **Chemotherapy treatment.** Thrombocytopaenia secondary to chemotherapy or radiotherapy can cause a bleeding diathesis. Carboplatin is commonly used in chemotherapy regimens in the treatment of ovarian cancer. The dose-limiting toxicity is myelosuppression: anaemia and thrombocytopaenia are more common than leucopaenia. The platelet nadir after treatment with carboplatin occurs between days 14 and 17. It is unusual to develop significant bleeding problems until platelet counts fall to $10–20 \times 10^9/l$ or less, although the presence of other factors, such as infection or drugs affecting platelet function, may result in bleeding when platelet levels are higher than this.

3   **Metastatic disease.** Other potential causes of bleeding in patients with gynaecological cancer are thrombocytopaenia secondary to marrow infiltration or impaired hepatic synthesis of coagulation factors secondary to extensive liver metastases. Both of these are unusual patterns of spread in the common histological types of gynaecological cancers.

4 **Vitamin K deficiency**. This may also be a contributing causal factor arising from poor dietary intake or biliary obstruction.

5 **Disseminated intravascular coagulation (DIC)**. This is common in cancer patients and may contribute both to clotting and bleeding problems. Acute, severe DIC generally leads to low levels of coagulation factors and hence bleeding.

6 **Adverse drug effects**. Use of anticoagulants and drugs with antiplatelet activity, such as NSAIDS, dipyridamole and clopidogrel, may also be a cause for bleeding.

Assessment of bleeding problems

Important points in the history

Bleeding is a distressing problem and patients will usually report episodes of obvious frank blood loss, such as vaginal bleeding. Attempts to estimate the amount is useful by asking about how frequently pads or tampons need changing and the duration of bleeding. The colour of blood loss and presence of clots may also help give some indication of the briskness with which bleeding is occurring. Provoking factors should be sought.

Necrotic tumour masses not only bleed but also may become infected, so that the patient reports a dark vaginal discharge. Specific enquiry about other less obvious manifestations of bleeding should be made as the development of unprovoked bruises or petechial rashes, may indicate low platelet counts. Discolouration of the urine may be due to haematuria, but is not always recognized by patients as such. Enquiry about recent chemotherapy or radiotherapy treatments and a detailed drug history are both essential.

Patients should also be asked their views on blood transfusion, as some religious groups forbid this.

Important points on examination

When a patient is bleeding acutely, with continuous brisk bleeding, regular pulse and blood pressure recordings are needed to assess and monitor her cardiovascular stability. If it is not clear from where bleeding is arising, inspection of the vagina and rectum should be done followed by a digital examination. An important exception to this is patients who are undergoing chemotherapy, where rectal or vaginal examination should not be performed if it is possible that the patient is neutropenic. Under these circumstances the risk of bacteraemia provoked by an intimate examination is best avoided unless the specific clinical situation dictates otherwise.

Inspection of the patient's limbs, trunk, and chest for bruising or petechial rashes is necessary if bleeding is thought to be secondary to a bleeding diathesis.

The patient's psychological state should also be assessed, as some patients will feel very anxious and frightened, and this will need to be taken into account when investigations or treatments are being planned.

Possible investigations

Investigations will be guided by clinical situation and the patient's wishes. Useful blood tests include a full blood count, clotting screen, serum urea electrolyte, and liver function tests. Where indicated, a sample should be sent for cross-matching, or group and save if transfusion is likely to be required in the future, avoiding the need for a repeat venepuncture later.

Who else may help?

Gynaecological surgical colleagues will be able to advise on possible surgical interventions or local treatments for bleeding. Medical and clinical oncologists will advise on the scope for further radiotherapy or chemotherapy treatment that may alleviate bleeding problems. Haematologists can advise on the possible aetiology and further investigation of bleeding problems and available medical therapy.

Management of bleeding problems

When managing a patient with advanced gynaecological cancer who has a bleeding problem, first consider her individual circumstances taking account of her general physical state, her likely prognosis, and options for further palliative anticancer treatments. Decisions will need to be guided by her views, especially if interventional measures to control bleeding are proposed.

Correcting drug-induced anticoagulation is an important first consideration when patients are on warfarin or heparin. The clinical picture and the level of INR or APTT will guide the method used. Any drugs with antiplatelet effects should be stopped.

Drug therapy

For many patients with very advanced cancer, drug therapy provides an acceptable approach to controlling bleeding. The most useful drugs are tranexamic acid and aminocaproic acid, which prevent lysis of fibrin clots by an inhibitory action on plasmin.

Tranexamic acid is more potent than aminocaproic acid and has a longer duration of activity and a lower incidence of side-effects. Both drugs are used in palliative care practice. Aminocaproic acid requires more frequent dosing (a loading dose of 5 g followed by 1–1.5 g every hour) to maintain its inhibitory effect on fibrinolysis, whereas tranexamic acid 1–1.5 g can be given two to four times daily. In patients with renal impairment it is necessary to reduce the dose and extend the dose intervals of both drugs because they are excreted renally.

It is generally recommended that therapy with tranexamic acid or aminocaproic acid should be continued until clinical symptoms resolve. In a study of 16 cancer patients, tranexamic acid was continued for a further 7 days on an empirical basis with good effect.[10] In the same study it was found that 15 of 16 patients experienced improvement, 14 having complete cessation of bleeding. The average time to improvement was 2 days and the average time to bleeding cessation was 4 days. Recurrence of bleeding after stopping treatment occurred in three patients, one of whom had abandoned therapy after one dose because of side-effects.

The main side-effects of tranexamic acid and aminocaproic acid are dose-related gastro-intestinal ones (nausea, vomiting, and diarrhoea).

Thrombo-embolism is a theoretical complication of treatment with fibrinolytic inhibitors but there is very little reported evidence of this happening in practice. Another reported contra-indication is massive haematuria because of concerns that intravesical clot formation may prove troublesome. In clinical practice, clot formation in the bladder may already be a problem when bleeding is heavy. In the previously cited study, four patients in whom this was the case benefited from tranexamic acid therapy, and it was postulated that this could be due to coagulation being initiated at the epithelial surface of the bladder.

Topical use of fibrinolytic inhibitors may also be useful; for example, by application to superficial fungating tumours, or by rectal or bladder instillation.

Ethamyslate is thought to work by correcting abnormal platelet adhesion. It is less often used than tranexamic acid. In theory ethamsylate could be used in conjunction with antifibrinolytic agents.

Antibiotic treatment is indicated when patients have offensive bloodstained vaginal discharge, as successful treatment of infection may help stop the bleeding.

Other medical therapy

There are several specialist techniques or interventions for dealing with significant vaginal bleeding secondary to advanced gynaecological cancer. Some patients will be too frail to undergo them.

Torrential distressing vaginal bleeding may require vaginal packing, whilst more definitive treatments are being considered.

Radiotherapy can be helpful: it is most appropriate for those patients who are relatively fit and whose life-expectancy is measured in months rather than days or weeks. Treatment regimens vary. In one recent study, single fractions of 10 Gy to the whole pelvis (repeated two to three times at 4-week intervals) was reported to give good symptomatic relief of vaginal bleeding in 90% of patients with advanced cancer of the body of uterus or cervix.[11] A dose-response effect was observed. Patients who had previously received radiotherapy were limited to one treatment. Acute toxicity was mild and only experienced by half of the patients as mild gastro-intestinal symptoms. For those patients who survived more than 10 months, and in whom two or three treatments had been given, serious late bowel complications occurred in 10%, which is an important factor to consider when selecting patients.

Other rarely indicated, but sometimes appropriate, methods of dealing with life-threatening haemorrhage include percutaneous transcatheter arterial embolization using particles, coils, or balloons, and laparoscopic ligature of the hypogastric artery.

Important palliative care points

For some patients bleeding is a persistent or recurrent problem despite efforts to control it. Good nursing care and detailed attention to physical comfort will be extremely important for these patients Reassurance and a calm approach to episodes of brisk bleeding will be helpful.

A plan should be in place for dealing with the possibility of a massive brisk haemorrhage as a terminal event. Under these circumstances the patient should not be left alone, and medication to provide sedation should be given as soon as possible if distress is evident. Anticipation of such events will mean that 'as required' medication (such as midazolam 5–10 mg to be given by subcutaneous injection) is already prescribed on the patients drug chart allowing nursing staff to take action quickly if needed.

It is useful to have green or dark blue towels or sheets available for a patient who is likely to bleed. This practical measure can reduce the alarming visual impact of fresh bleeding on patients and carers. Blood staining appears less dramatic when toned down by a dark background material.

References

1 Trousseau, A. (1865). Phlegmasia alba dolens. In *Clinique medicale de l'Hotel-Dieu de Paris*, vol.3, pp. 654–712. J.B. Ballière et Fils, Paris.

2 Walsh, J. J., Bonnar, J., and Wright, F. W. (1974). A study of pulmonary embolism and deep leg vein thrombosis after major gynaecologic surgery using labelled fibrinogen, phlebography and lung scanning. *J Obstet Gynaecol Br Commonw*, **31**, 311–6.

3 von Tempelhoff, G. F., Dietrich, M., Niemann, F., Schneider, D., Hommel, G., and Heilmann, L. (1997). Blood coagulation and thrombosis in patients with ovarian malignancy. *Thromb Haemost*, **77**, 456–61.

4 Wells, P. S., Hirsch, J., Anderson, D. R., Lensing, A. W., Foster, G., Kearon, C. *et al.* (1995). Accuracy of clinical assessment of deep vein thrombosis. *Lancet*, **345**, 1326–30.

5 ten Wolde, M., Kraaijenhagen, R. A., Prins, M. H., and Buller, H. R. (2002). The clinical usefulness of D-Dimer testing in cancer patients with suspected deep venous thrombosis. *Arch Int Med*, **162**, 1880–4.

6 Johnson, M. J. and Sherry, K. (1997). How do palliative physicians manage venous thrombembolism. *Pall Med*, **11**, 462–68.

7 Johnson, M. J. (1997). Bleeding, clotting and cancer. *Clin Oncol*, **9**, 294–301.

8 Oden, A. and Fahlen, M. (2002). Oral anticoagulation and risk of death: a medical record linkage study. *BMJ*, **32**, 1073–5.

9 Evans, T. R., Mansi, J. L., and Bevan, D. H. (1996). Trousseau's syndrome in association with ovarian carcinoma. *Cancer*, **77**, 2544–9.

10 Dean, A. and Tuffin, P. (1997). Fibrinolytic inhibitors for cancer associated bleeding problems. *J Pain Symptom Manage*, **13**, 20–4.

11 Onsrud, M., Hagen, B., and Stricert, T. (2001). 10-Gy single fraction pelvic irradiation for palliation and life prolongation in patients with cancer of the cervix and corpus uteri. *Gynecol Oncol*, **82**, 167–71.

Chapter 10

The management of ascites

Karen Bowen, Jay R. Thomas, and
Charles F. von Gunten

Summary

Ascites, the accumulation of fluid in the abdomen, is common in patients with epithelial malignancies such as ovarian and endometrial carcinomas. It may be responsible for, or contribute to, multiple debilitating symptoms. Its formation may be a direct result of a malignant process or secondary to an unrelated co-morbidity. Because the pathophysiology of fluid collection varies, treatment strategies differ. Understanding and clinically distinguishing the mechanisms responsible for ascites are imperative for rational management.

Assessment of people with ascites requires close attention to all domains of patient care, including physical, psychological, social, and practical issues. History and physical examination (including specific manoeuvres) are often adequate to diagnose ascites. When equivocal, imaging can confirm the presence of even small amounts of fluid. Diagnostic paracentesis and calculation of the serum–ascites albumin gradient (SAAG, Fig. 10.1) is essential to determine aetiology and guide treatment strategy.

The goals for patient care must be considered before specific choices for managing ascites are made. Every intervention has associated burdens and benefits that need to be considered and discussed. Systemic chemotherapy or intraperitoneal treatment with chemotherapeutic or biologic agents may be effective for patients with ascites due to a responsive malignancy. Ascites with a SAAG $\geq$ 1.1 g/dl may respond to dietary restrictions and/or diuretics. Therapeutic paracentesis is often required. Surgical procedures such as peritoneovenous shunts or implanted abdominal catheters may be beneficial in patients requiring serial paracentesis.

Summary of sources of evidence

The evidence base for this review comes from published works in the English language identified through a search of the MEDLINE database since 1966.

Background concepts

Epidemiology

Only 10% of patients who have ascites will have a malignancy as the primary cause. Epithelial malignancies, particularly ovarian, endometrial, breast, colon, gastric, and pancreatic carcinomas, cause over 80% of malignant ascites. The remaining 20% are due to malignancies of unknown origin. In one study, Runyon has shown that 53.3% of malignant ascites is associated with peritoneal carcinomatosis, 13.3% is associated with massive liver metastases, 13.3% is associated with peritoneal carcinomatosis and massive liver metastases, 13.3% is associated with hepatocellular carcinoma with portal hypertension, and 6.7% is associated with chylous ascites.[1]

In general, the presence of ascites portends a poor prognosis. The mean survival in patients with malignant ascites is generally less than 4 months. However, with ascites due to a malignancy that is relatively sensitive to chemotherapy, such as newly diagnosed ovarian cancer, the mean survival may improve significantly to 32 and 58 weeks, respectively.

Pathophysiology

Multiple and complex mechanisms are responsible for malignant ascites. Liver metastases can cause hepatic venous obstruction and result in portal hypertension. Increased portal pressure leads to transudation of fluid across the splanchnic bed into the abdominal cavity. The ascites of peritoneal carcinomatosis accumulates via a different mechanism. Tumour cells on the peritoneal surface directly interfere with normal venous and lymphatic drainage, causing fluid to 'leak' into the abdomen. A humoral vascular permeability factor that allows exudation of fluid from the peritoneal vessels has also been identified.[2] Chylous ascites can result from the lymphatic obstruction commonly seen in lymphoma. In cancer patients, diminished intravascular oncotic pressure resulting from hypo-albuminaemia may exacerbate ascites accumulation. Any of these mechanisms may be complicated by the abnormal sodium and fluid retention of co-morbid cirrhosis or congestive heart failure. Other co-morbid causes of non-malignant ascites are tuberculosis, nephrogenic ascites related to haemodialysis, pancreatic disease, portal vein thrombosis, pericardial disease, and nephrotic syndrome.

Serum–ascites albumin gradient

The serum–ascites albumin gradient (SAAG) is helpful in discriminating between mechanisms of ascites because it directly correlates with portal pressure.[3] It is calculated by subtracting the ascitic fluid albumin concentration

$$SAAG = [\text{Serum albumin (g/dl)}]-[\text{ascitic albumin (g/dl)}]$$
$$SAAG \geq 1.1 \Rightarrow \Uparrow \text{portal pressures} \Rightarrow \text{diuretic response}$$

Fig. 10.1 Serum–ascites albumin gradient.

from the serum albumin concentration (Fig. 10.1). Patients with a SAAG of 1.1 g/dl or more have ascites that is due, at least in part, to increased portal pressures. Patients with a SAAG of less than 1.1 g/dl do not have portal hypertension. These correlations are accurate to 97%. The SAAG is superior to, and has superseded, the exudate/transudate characterizations that are based solely on ascitic fluid protein concentrations. In general, a high SAAG predicts diuretic responsiveness. One exception is the nephrotic syndrome where although the SAAG is low, it is typically responsive to diuretics.

Assessment

History

Patients with ascites may complain of multiple debilitating symptoms, including dyspnea, fatigue, anorexia, early satiety, nausea, vomiting, pain, or diminished exercise tolerance. Recent weight gain, increases in abdominal girth (with or without protrusion of the umbilicus), a sensation of fullness or bloating, and early satiety suggest the presence of abdominal fluid accumulation. Some people simply describe a vague generalized abdominal discomfort or a feeling of heaviness with ambulation. Increased intra-abdominal pressure can produce oesophageal reflux symptoms. Delayed gastric emptying may prompt complaints of indigestion, nausea, and vomiting. As disease progresses, an increasing accumulation of abdominal fluid can severely compromise quality of life and challenge patients and caregivers.

Careful ongoing assessment of all domains of patient care is essential, including physical, psychological, social, and practical issues. For example, abdominal distention and concurrent oedema may dramatically affect body image and mobility. Social interactions may be affected and patients may become isolated. Mood may become altered. Therapeutic interventions may actually increase burdens to the patient and caregivers. Frequent urination may disturb sleep or sociability. Bulky external catheters may be awkward or uncomfortable.

Effective management of these complex issues requires an ongoing assessment of the goals of care, so that recommendations will meet the overall needs of the patient and family. An interdisciplinary approach to assessment and management will provide the best results.

Physical examination

The physical examination for ascites includes inspection for bulging flanks, percussion for flank dullness, a test for shifting dullness, and a test for a fluid wave. Jugular venous distension should be assessed as it may indicate a potentially reversible cardiac cause of ascites.

The weight of ascitic fluid will cause abdominal flanks to bulge when supine. Ascites may be distinguished from adipose tissue by percussing for dullness. To detect flank dullness in the supine patient, approximately 1500 ml of fluid must be present. Further evidence of ascites is demonstrated by noting that the dullness shifts upward toward the umbilicus when the patient is turned partially toward the side that has been percussed (shifting dullness).

The elicitation of a fluid wave may also help to confirm the diagnosis. An assistant places the medial edges of both hands firmly down the midline of the abdomen to block transmission of a wave through subcutaneous fat. The examiner places his/her hands on the flanks and then taps one flank sharply while simultaneously using the fingertips of the opposite hand to feel for an impulse transmitted through the ascites to the other flank. This test is 90% specific, but only 62% sensitive.

Several additional aspects of the physical examination may also be helpful. Umbilical, abdominal, or inguinal hernias, lower extremity oedema, or abdominal wall venous engorgement may be present if ascites is severe. An enlarged liver may be ballottable. The umbilicus may be flattened or slightly protuberant.

Diagnostic imaging

A plain radiograph of the abdomen may demonstrate a hazy or ground-glass pattern. Ultrasound or computed tomography will identify as little as 100 ml of free fluid, and will be helpful if loculation is present.

Diagnostic paracentesis

A diagnostic paracentesis of 10–20 ml of fluid will confirm the presence of ascites. More importantly, determining the SAAG will indicate whether portal hypertension is present or not and will direct therapy.

Paracentesis may be safely performed in two locations. The first is over the linea alba, which is typically avascular, 2 cm below the umbilicus. The second location is lateral to the edge of the rectus sheath, 2 cm superior and medial to the anterior iliac spine. Previous surgery in the area of the procedure increases the possibility that bowel may be adherent to the abdominal wall.

Ultrasonography may be performed if surgical scarring is present, fluid is difficult to obtain, or loculation is suspected.

To minimize the risk of leaking fluid following the procedure, the Z technique is performed. After careful cleansing and local anaesthetizing, a 2-inch, 20-gauge angiocatheter is attached to a 20-ml syringe. The skin is displaced 2 cm relative to the deep fascia. To avoid trapping omentum or bowel against the needle tip, a small amount of negative pressure is intermittently applied through the syringe while the needle is slowly advanced and ascitic fluid is obtained. When the needle is withdrawn the facial planes will overlap to prevent fluid leakage. Fluid colour should be noted. White milky fluid is characteristic of chylous ascites. Bloody fluid is almost always malignant in origin, but may be due to abdominal tuberculosis. Initial bloody fluid that clears is more likely related to procedural trauma.

In addition to measuring ascitic albumin concentration to determine the SAAG, several other diagnostic tests may be useful. Cytologic analysis is the most specific test to demonstrate malignant ascites. It is about 97% sensitive with peritoneal carcinomatosis, but is poor in detecting other types of malignant ascites. Cell counts with a differential are useful in the presumptive diagnosis of bacterial peritonitis, particularly if the neutrophil count is greater than 250 cells per ml. A Gram stain and culture should be performed if infection is suspected. Inoculation of ascites directly into blood culture bottles increases the sensitivity of detecting infection up to 85%.

Management

General considerations

Interventions for ascites management in the supportive or palliative care setting should generally be reserved for patients who are symptomatic. The goals for patient care must be considered before specific choices for managing ascites are made. The prognosis, expected response to management of the underlying conditions, and preferences for treatment should first be established with the patient and family before any treatment plan is instituted. Every intervention has associated burdens and benefits that need to be realistically considered and discussed.

Chemotherapy and biological agents

Palliative goals are to minimize symptoms and optimize quality of life without the expectation that the underlying cause can be cured. For patients with ascites due to a malignancy that is responsive to chemotherapy (like ovarian cancer), systemic chemotherapy may be an effective palliative management strategy. Early clinical trials for treatment of malignant ascites with intraperitoneal chemotherapeutic or biological agents have yielded mixed results. Their overall efficacy and role in both curative and palliative care remains to be determined.

Sodium and fluid balance

Since ascites fluid due to portal hypertension is in equilibrium with total body fluid, efforts to restrict salt and affect fluid balance with diuretics are often successful in this group. Malignant ascites may or may not be responsive to these efforts depending on its cause.[4] In cases of massive hepatic metastasis, portal hypertension is present and the resulting malignant ascites is responsive to salt restriction and diuretics, but it may not always be appropriate: this depends on the goals of care. In peritoneal carcinomatosis and chylous ascites, however, there is no portal hypertension and the ascites is not in equilibrium with total body fluid. Consequently, dietary restriction and diuretics may be of little use. Their injudicious use may result in intravascular volume depletion, diminished renal perfusion, azotaemia, hypotension, and fatigue. Since many cancer patients have complex factors contributing to their ascites, the serum–ascites albumin gradient may be critically helpful in determining the management plan (Table 10.1).

Table 10.1 Causes of ascites and diuretic responsiveness

Cause of ascites	SAAG	Predicted diuretic response
Peritoneal carcinomatosis	Low (≤1.1 g/dl)	No
Massive hepatic metastasis	High (≥1.1 g/dl)	Yes
Mixed ascites (i.e. cirrhosis plus infection or cancer)	High (≥1.1 g/dl)	Yes
Portal vein thrombosis	High (≥1.1 g/dl)	Yes
Veno-occlusive disease	High (≥1.1 g/dl)	Yes
Bowel obstruction/infarction	Low (≤1.1 g/dl)	No
Fulminant hepatic failure	High (≥1.1 g/dl)	Yes
Cirrhosis	High (≥1.1 g/dl)	Yes
Cardiac ascites	High (≥1.1 g/dl)	Yes
Pancreatic or biliary ascites (without cirrhosis)	Low (≤1.1 g/dl)	No
Nephrotic syndrome	Low (≤1.1 g/dl)	Yes

Dietary management

When portal hypertension is present, dietary management may be helpful. Symptoms may be improved with sodium restriction. Limiting sodium intake to 88 mmol or 2 gm per day (equivalent to 5 gm of sodium chloride per day) is an attainable goal for a motivated patient but does make food less palatable. Considering a patient's goals of care, it may be better to liberalize the sodium intake and control ascites through other methods. These patients are also prone to develop dilutional hyponatraemia. In patients with advanced disease whose treatment goals are purely palliative, the typical fluid restriction to 1 l per day is usually intolerably burdensome. Serum sodium levels gradually dropping to as low as 120 mmol per l may be well-tolerated and rarely dictate restrictive intervention.

Diuretics

Diuretic therapy is useful for some patients, particularly those with a component of portal hypertension (high SAAG). Goals with diuretic therapy are to achieve a slow and gradual diuresis that does not exceed the capacity for mobilization of ascitic fluid. Only enough fluid should be mobilized to promote comfort. In patients with ascites and oedema, oedema will act as a fluid reservoir to buffer the effects of a rapid contraction of plasma volume. A net diuresis of approximately 1 l per day is safe. Symptomatic orthostatic hypotension from intravascular volume contraction is more likely to occur in patients without oedema. In this group, a net diuresis of 500 ml per day is more reasonable. Overly aggressive diuretic therapy in patients with ascites due to cirrhosis has been associated with hepatorenal syndrome and death. There are no published reports of hepatorenal syndrome associated with malignant ascites.

The renin–angiotensin–aldosterone system is activated in patients with ascites for whom diuretics may be helpful. Therefore, the initial diuretic of choice is a distal tubule aldosterone antagonist. Sprinolactone started at 100 mg per day and titrated to effect or maximum dose (400 mg per day) is often useful (Table 10.2). Amiloride is faster acting, and may be used as an alternative if painful gynaecomastia develops. These diuretics are relatively potassium sparing, and patients should be advised to avoid potassium salt substitutes.

Diuretics acting upon different segments of the nephron may produce a synergistic response. If response to spironolactone is suboptimal, a loop diuretic may be added. This combination may affect a more rapid diuresis while maintaining potassium homeostasis. A ratio of 100 mg of spironolactone

Table 10.2 Diuretics

Diuretic	Major site of action	Dosage range
Spironolactone	Distal tubule	100–400 mg/day
Amiloride	Distal tubule	10–40 mg/day
Triamterene	Distal tubule	100–300 mg/day
Furosemide	Loop of Henle	40–160 mg/day
Ethacrynic acid	Loop of Henle	50–200 mg/day

to 40 mg of furosemide is recommended, with further adjustments to maintain normokalaemia. The dosages can be increased in parallel until the goals of therapy have been attained (not to exceed maximal doses), or until therapy is limited by side-effects.

The sequential addition of diuretics is usually recommended. Although there is no evidence to support the combined use of multiple types of diuretics at the beginning of therapy, this may be an appropriate management strategy in a population with limited life expectancy and distressing symptoms. Precious time may be gained by starting with a spironolactone/furosemide combination in the ratios described above.

Non-steroidal anti-inflammatory medications can alter glomerular filtration and inhibit prostaglandin promotion of sodium and water excretion. Their discontinuation may increase diuretic efficacy. If these drug interactions have been minimized, salt intake is appropriate, and there is no response to maximal diuretic therapy, the ascites is considered refractory.

The possible burdens of diuretic therapy

Diuretic therapy may be excessively burdensome in patients with limited mobility, urinary tract outflow symptoms such as hesitancy and frequency, poor appetite and poor oral intake, or complex polypharmacy. Injudicious diuretics can result in incontinence with attendant self-esteem and skin care issues, sleep deprivation from frequent urination, fatigue from hyponatraemia and/or hypokalaemia, and falls from postural hypotension.

Therapeutic paracentesis

In the patient with refractory ascites, paracentesis may be the only therapeutic modality that is effective. The symptom response is much faster than when diuretics are used alone. If the ascites is in equilibrium with the systemic circulation, as is the case with portal hypertension, there is a risk of haemodynamic compromise. Colloid plasma volume expansion (e.g. 6–8 g albumin/l ascites removed) has been used to avoid this complication, but its use remains controversial. Further studies may elucidate under what circumstances colloid is and is not indicated. Although albumin is expensive, it is not known to cause harm. Large-volume therapeutic paracentesis ($\geqslant$5 l) with concurrent colloid infusion is a simple procedure and is associated with minimal morbidity or mortality. Practitioners may opt to use colloid for large-volume paracentesis of ascites due to portal hypertension until more definitive guidelines exist.

Implanted external catheters

Tenckhoff or other implanted abdominal catheters may be beneficial for selected patients who require repeated large-volume paracentesis for comfort and whose prognosis warrants an invasive procedure.[5] Under local anaesthesia, an externally draining catheter is surgically placed in the peritoneal cavity. This drain can be conveniently accessed intermittently by physicians or nurses, or even by trained family members. The comfort advantage of the smaller, less obtrusive devices is offset by tendency for occlusion. To date, there are no studies comparing implanted catheters with serial paracentesis in patients with either cirrhotic or malignant ascites. Complications such as cellulitis, peritonitis, and asymptomatic culture-positive ascites have been reported. With no guidance from the literature, use of implanted catheters must be individualized.

Peritoneovenous shunts

Surgically placed peritoneovenous shunts (LeVeen, Denver, and others) have been used for management of malignant and non-malignant ascites. The 30–60-min procedure is performed under local anaesthesia. These shunts drain ascites from the peritoneal space via a one-way valve into the thoracic venous system. Unfortunately, the rate of complications is high, including shunt occlusion, heart failure due to fluid overload, infection, and disseminated intravascular coagulation. In malignant ascites, studies have found no improvement in survival or quality of life. Thus, although there may be specific cases where peritoneovenous shunting is advantageous, serial paracentesis remains the first line therapy.

Transjugular intrahepatic portosystemic shunt (TIPS)

The transjugular intrahepatic portosystemic shunt is a procedure performed by interventional radiologists that creates a side-to-side shunt that effectively relieves portal hypertension. For patients with cirrhosis and refractory ascites with relatively good hepatic and renal function, TIPS is considered the treatment of choice. However, shunt malfunction rates of up to 40% have been reported. In two cases of malignant portal and hepatic vein occlusion, TIPS improved ascites and quality of life.[6] As with any palliative management option, the decision to pursue invasive surgical procedures is dependent on the patient's goals and the disease context.

References

1 Runyon, B. A., Hoefs, J. C., and Morgan, T. R. (1988). Ascitic fluid analysis in malignancy-related ascites. *Hepatology*, 8, 1104–9.

2 Senger, D. R., Galli, S. J., Dvorak, A. M., Perruzzi, C. A., Harvey, V. S., and Dvorak, H. F. (1983). Tumour cells secrete a vascular permeability factor that promotes accumulation of ascites fluid. *Science*, 219, 983–5.

3 Hoefs, J. C. (1983). Serum protein concentration and portal pressure determine the ascitic fluid protein concentration in patients with chronic liver disease. *J Lab Clin Med*, 102, 260–73.

4 Pockros, P. J., Esrason, K. T., Nguyen, C., Duque, J., and Woods, S. (1992). Mobilization of malignant ascites with diuretics is dependent on ascitic fluid characteristics. *Gastroenterology*, 103, 1302–6.

5 Barnett, T. D. and Rubins, J. (2002). Placement of a permanent tunneled peritoneal drainage catheter for palliation of malignant ascites: a simplified percutaneous approach. *J Vasc Interv Radiol*, 13, 379–83.

6 Burger, J. A., Ochs, A., Wirth, K., Berger, D. P., Mertelsmann, R., Engelhardt, R. *et al.* (1997). The transjugular stent implantation for the treatment of malignant portal and hepatic vein obstruction in cancer patients. *Ann Oncol*, 8, 200–2.

Chapter 11

The management of urinary tract obstruction in advanced pelvic disease

Sarah K. Richards and Alastair W. S. Ritchie

Introduction

Malignant disease, invading the genito-urinary system, can produce an array of problematic and distressing symptoms, as well as life-threatening biochemical abnormalities. The possible causes of urinary obstruction are numerous. Ureteric obstruction can be caused by diseases of the urinary tract itself but may also be affected by diseases of the retroperitoneum, the gastro-intestinal tract, the female reproductive system, and a variety of vascular pathologies. Urinary tract obstruction can be iatrogenic in origin and follow surgery and radiotherapy to structures close to the ureter. This chapter concentrates on the management of patients with obstruction of the urinary tract as a result of advanced gynaecological malignancy. Obstructive uropathy is seen commonly in pelvic, retroperitoneal, and abdominal malignancies. The management approach for these patients will depend upon the site of obstruction, the patient's general condition and prognosis.

Bladder outlet obstruction is seen in advanced cancers of the cervix, vulva, bladder, prostate, or urethra. Ureteric obstruction may result from para-aortic nodal metastases from ovarian, breast, gastro-intestinal, prostatic, or bladder primaries. Intra-abdominal lymphomas or sarcomas are other possible causes. The patient with a past history of malignancy should not be assumed to have malignancy as the cause of obstruction uropathy, although this is more likely in advanced gynaecological malignancy than some other cancers. Benign disease, including calculi and retroperitoneal fibrosis, should be included in the differential diagnosis. This chapter concentrates on the practical aspects of symptom control in this group of patients with an emphasis on simple, problem-orientated management. The management of such patients can be difficult and at times controversial. Decisions to instigate invasive or aggressive management should be made for each patient as an individual, and only when the stage of disease, life-expectancy, and the patient's wishes and goals have been carefully considered.

Incidence

Pelvic malignant neoplasms represent the second most common cause of extrinsic obstructive uropathy in women—the gravid uterus is the commonest cause. Squamous carcinoma of the cervix is best known for its propensity to involve the urinary tract. Approximately 2500 women die each year in the United Kingdom of cervical carcinoma, and the most common cause of death amongst these women is urinary obstruction, which is responsible in at least 50% of cases. Ureteric obstruction usually occurs at the vesico-ureteric junction due to external compression either due to tumour bulk or nodal metastases. Ureteric involvement in cervical carcinoma is associated with a grave prognosis. The 5-year survivals for patients with and without ureteric obstruction have been shown to be approximately 14% and 50%, respectively.[1] This has led to patients with ureteric involvement being placed into an advanced stage group (IIIB).

Bladder carcinoma is the second most common female cause of malignant obstruction after cervical carcinoma. Transitional cell carcinoma can be multi-focal and may involve the urothelium from renal calyces to urethra.

Obstructive uropathy has a greater incidence in men after 60 years, reflecting the increasing incidence of prostatic disease with advancing age. The majority of obstructive problems are secondary to benign prostatic hypertrophy but an increasing proportion, are due to malignant disease. Prostatic carcinoma may spread locally to involve the bladder neck, trigone, and ureteric orifices. Lymphatic spread may result in bulky nodal deposits, causing external compression of the ureters higher up in their course.

Other malignancies may also cause obstructive uropathy by metastasis—an overall frequency of 1% has been quoted from a major autopsy series. Rare childhood tumours may also cause uraemia by obstruction. These include pelvic neurofibromas, and Wilm's tumours, which can cause upper tract obstruction in 70% of patients.

Patho-physiology of obstructive uropathy

The patho-physiology of urinary tract obstruction is complex and not yet fully understood. The majority of animal and human models studied in a laboratory setting have focused on complete urinary tract obstruction over a 24-h period only. The major acute changes seen are as follows:

- A progressive rise in intra-luminal pressure.
- Renal tract dilatation proximal to the site of obstruction.

◆ Increased afferent blood flow to the kidney caused by dilatation of afferent arterioles. This hyperaemic response appears to be the result of an intrinsic renal mechanism probably mediated by the macula densa.

◆ Impaired urinary acidification predominantly in the collecting duct. This is due to an inability to create a negative luminal voltage within the nephron into which it can secrete hydrogen ions, probably due to H-ATPase damage on the apical membrane.

◆ Reduced capacity to either concentrate or dilute urine thus urine osmolality in complete obstruction approaches that of plasma.

◆ Reduced re-absorption of Na^+ and excretion of K^+ at many sites throughout the length of the nephron—predominantly due to down-regulation of transporter proteins. It remains unknown how obstruction directly affects the activity of these proteins.

◆ Increased anaerobic respiration resulting in reduced ATP levels in tissues throughout the body.

◆ Thinning of the renal parenchyma, which results in a reduced functional mass over time.

Obstruction resulting from malignant disease is usually of slower onset and may modify the changes outlined above.

Assessment of the patient

History and examination

A careful history and examination can yield a diagnosis of acute urinary tract obstruction and the level at which it may have occurred. However, in patients with an insidious onset of obstruction, symptoms may be less marked.

An overall assessment of the patient is crucial in establishing volume status. Dry mucous membranes, reduced skin turgor, reduced capillary refill, and postural blood pressure changes are seen in 'volume-depleted' patients. Alternatively, a raised jugular venous pressure, pulmonary basal crackles, and ankle/sacral oedema suggests fluid overload. Careful examination may also reveal pallor pointing to anaemia and drowsiness and irritability suggesting uraemia.

Unilateral ureteric obstruction

Unilateral obstruction will classically present with unilateral loin pain thought to result from stretching of the renal capsule. The severity of pain may correlate with rate of obstruction and urine output. Pain is often most severe after the patient has drunk a large volume of fluid. A palpable or ballottable loin

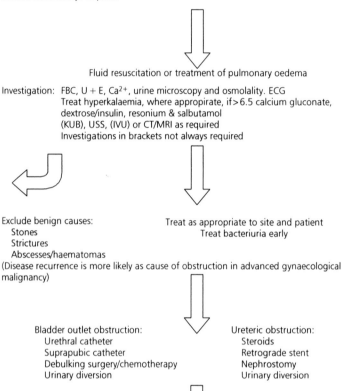

HISTORY AND EXAMINATION

Full assessment should include complete history and discussion with the patient about her goals and priorities. Aggressive treatment of urinary obstruction is not always appropirate, careful assessment is always required

Fluid resuscitation or treatment of pulmonary oedema

Investigation: FBC, U + E, Ca^{2+}, urine microscopy and osmolality. ECG
Treat hyperkalaemia, where appropirate, if > 6.5 calcium gluconate, dextrose/insulin, resonium & salbutamol
(KUB), USS, (IVU) or CT/MRI as required
Investigations in brackets not always required

Exclude benign causes:
  Stones
  Strictures
  Abscesses/haematomas
(Disease recurrence is more likely as cause of obstruction in advanced gynaecological malignancy)

Treat as appropriate to site and patient
Treat bacteriuria early

Bladder outlet obstruction:
  Urethral catheter
  Suprapubic catheter
  Debulking surgery/chemotherapy
  Urinary diversion

Ureteric obstruction:
  Steroids
  Retrograde stent
  Nephrostomy
  Urinary diversion

Treat post-obstructive diuresis aggressively
Replace urine output with 0.45% or 0.9% N. Saline
Monitor U + E closely and replace K$^+$ early
Wean IV fluids after 24 h

Fig. 11.1

mass may indicate marked hydronephrosis but is rare as a clinical sign. Episodes of oliguria may alternate with episodes of polyuria.

Bilateral ureteric obstruction

Bilateral ureteric obstruction can produce similar but bilateral symptoms or may be silent in its presentation.

Bladder outlet obstruction

Bladder outlet obstruction results in low abdominal pain and a strong desire to void if it is of acute onset. Total anuria may be seen. Once again, these symptoms may not be seen if the rate of obstruction is slow. Slower onset type symptoms that are classical include poor urinary stream, nocturia, nocturnal enuresis and post void dribbling. A history of recurrent urinary tract infections is common in patients with large residual urine volumes. A palpable mass and/or dullness to percussion in the suprapubic region may be due to a distended bladder. Digital rectal examination and/or vaginal examination is of paramount importance in these patients.

Investigations

Routine haematological and biochemical investigations are frequently abnormal in urinary tract obstruction. Biochemical measurements may show a raised serum creatinine, urea, and potassium. Derangements in serum sodium (Na), chloride (Cl) and bicarbonate (HCO_3) may also occur. A full blood count may reveal a raised white count indicative of supervening infection or, rarely, involvement of the urinary tract by haematological malignancies. Anaemia of chronic disease may also be seen in these patients, attributable to new urinary tract pathology or as a result of existing malignancy. Anaemia may also accompany chronic renal failure as a result of diminished erythropoietin secretion.

Urine microscopy is imperative. Microscopic haematuria may indicate tumour or calculus. The presence of white cells or bacteriuria should raise the possibility of pyelonephritis or stasis, respectively. Visible crystals should alert the clinician to nephrolithiasis. An ECG is indicated in patients with electrolyte imbalance, especially where there are abnormalities of serum potassium.

Urine osmolality can be a useful tool. In chronic renal damage a picture similar to acute tubular necrosis may be seen (Na >20 mEq/l and Osmolality <350 mOsm), whilst in acute obstruction a picture similar to pre-renal failure may be seen (Na <20 mEq/l and osmolality >500 mOsm).

Patients with co-existing malignancy have many reasons to have a benign cause for obstructive uropathy and this must be excluded. Lau et al.[2] reported that 55% of all ureteric strictures in patients with cervical carcinoma as being of benign aetiology. Uric acid nephropathy may be seen as a result of alkylating agents. Previous radiotherapy or instrumentation may cause benign strictures of the urinary tract, whilst surgery may result in abscesses, urinomas or haematomas, which may cause extra-luminal compression.

Plain abdominal film (KUB)

Approximately 90% of renal calculi are radio-opaque and may be seen located along the course of the ureter or bladder. This simple investigation may also give a rough idea as to size, position, and contour of the kidney(s). It is not always needed—for example, if the primary complaint is neuropathic pain.

Ultrasound

This investigation remains the preferred method of screening for urinary tract obstruction. It has a sensitivity and specificity for hydronephrosis in excess of 90%. It is safe, reliable, and cheap, and involves no radiation exposure. Ultrasonography of the kidney following prolonged urinary tract obstruction, will also detect renal parenchymal thinning. Whilst this technique remains a useful modality for screening, it is only able to approximate a level of obstruction. Further investigations are usually required to determine the exact anatomy and cause of the obstruction.

Intravenous urography (IVU)

This investigation has been superseded by ultrasound but remains a useful method for determining anatomy and the exact location of obstruction in the upper urinary tracts. With judicious use of delayed films, it can determine the site of obstruction except in very marked renal failure, where there may be insufficient renal tubular function to allow opacification. In recent obstruction, a prolonged nephron transit time will produce a characteristic delayed nephrogram. Calyces on an affected side will be seen to fill late and there will be proximal dilatation of the system down to the level of the occlusion. A post-micturition film can provide information about bladder emptying. This investigation does require intravenous administration of a potentially nephrotoxic iodine-based radio-opaque contrast and, in rare cases, causes severe allergic reactions. There are no disease-related contra-indications to IVU in gynaecological malignancy unlike myeloma where it should be used with great caution.

Antegrade pyelography

This invasive procedure requires percutaneous injection of contrast using a nephrostomy tube or needle into the renal pelvis under ultrasound control. It produces similar information to that obtained at IVU.

Cystoscopy and retrograde pyelography

This invasive technique allows examination of the urinary tract using contrast injected directly into the ureter. After performing diagnostic cystoscopy, a catheter (such a Chevassu 6F) is placed in the distal ureter. Contrast is injected into the ureter and an image intensifier is used to visualize the ureter and any obstructing lesion. In patients who are debilitated or immunosuppressed, such as oncology patients, there is a risk of causing bacteraemia from associated urinary tract sepsis. Prophylactic antibiotics can be given if there is any suspicion of infection in the urine drained from the bladder.

Pressure flow studies

Demonstration that high voiding pressures are required to attain an adequate urine flow is diagnostic of bladder outlet obstruction. Formal urodynamics and video cystography may be helpful adjuncts.

Computerised tomography (CT)

CT remains one of the best investigations for determining the exact cause of obstruction if it remains unclear following ultrasound or IVU. CT is especially good at identifying extrinsic causes of obstruction, such as nodal metastases or direct compression from a tumour primary in the abdomen. In oncology patients, it is particularly useful for establishing the extent and stage of disease, so an exact management strategy can be planned taking into account not only the current urinary tract obstruction, but also life-expectancy and any additional predicted problems.

MRI

This is the investigation of choice for detecting and assessing pelvic recurrence. In the UK where provision of MRI scanners is, at present, inadequate, CT and ultrasound may be the initial or only investigations used in a patient with malignancy.

Treating the problem

Conservative management

As much information as possible should be gathered before making crucial decisions on management. This needs to include open conversations involving the patient, family, and the multidisciplinary team, wherever possible. In advanced disease, symptom management may be all that is possible or reasonable. The patient's goals and the likelihood of successful treatment leading to a better quality of life need to be central considerations in patients with advanced cancer. An obstructed kidney in a patient with terminal disease may not require intervention if the opposite kidney is functioning. The combination of obstruction and infection usually demands intervention. It may not be possible to reach a definite decision until the patient's pain has been controlled and she has had some time to digest the seriousness of her predicament. Where doubt about the best course of action exists, and if the patient is in danger (due, for example, to electrolyte disturbance), it is usually better to go ahead with temporary drainage.

Medical

Fluid balance

Fluid balance must be optimized quickly: replacement should be started promptly if there is evidence of depletion and diuresis considered if the patient is overloaded. Careful clinical assessment of the patient (see previously) is usually sufficient to determine the state of hydration, although occasionally invasive central venous monitoring may be required. Catheterization is usually required to measure urine output accurately. There should be a low threshold for prophylactic antibiotic administration to prevent urinary tract sepsis when a catheter is to be passed. It is worth remembering that in cases of bilateral obstruction, urine output will not reflect fluid balance accurately. The rate of fluid resuscitation will vary from patient to patient, depending for example on the patient's age, body size, and the presence of cardiovascular and other disease. The type of fluid used will be determined by the degree of electrolyte disturbance. Normal saline (250–500 ml) may be given quickly as a bolus and further resuscitation fluid given according to reassessment. If the patient is obviously overloaded, 40–60 mg of frusemide intravenously or orally can be given but may not be effective in bilateral ureteric obstruction. In a case such as this, a glyceryl trinitrate (GTN) infusion will provide some symptomatic relief of pulmonary oedema until the obstruction is bypassed and an effective diuresis can be achieved.

Hyperkalaemia

There is need for urgent treatment of hyperkalaemia, where this is appropriate, if the potassium level is >6.5 or if ECG changes are seen (tented T waves, wide QRS complexes, or frequent escape complexes). For cardio protection, 10–20 ml of calcium gluconate (10%) IV should be administered. A bolus of dextrose insulin should be given (10–15 units of soluble insulin mixed with 50 ml of 50% dextrose should be given as an IV bolus). The patient should remain on a cardiac monitor until the serum potassium has returned to a reasonable level. Persistent hyperkalaemia may be treated with further boluses of dextrose/insulin or a continuous infusion according to frequent blood sugar measurements. Calcium resonium ion exchange resins may be used to remove excess potassium (15 g orally three times a day or 30 g as an enema). Salbutamol nebulizers may also be used as an adjunct (5 mg up to four hourly) but may cause a marked tremor and tachycardia. Potassium sparing diuretics (spironolactone) should be stopped, and fruits and juices should be avoided.

If hyperkalaemia remains marked despite this management (especially if accompanied by a significant acidosis pH <7.2), urgent dialysis or haemofiltration may be appropriate after careful thought and discussion. In very marked cases of acidosis (pH 7.1 or less), sodium bicarbonate as an emergency treatment may help other medical measures to reduce potassium more effectively but should be discussed with a renal physician.

Steroids

Several studies have prompted the use of corticosteroids in the management of malignant ureteric obstruction. One study describes the use of oral dexamethasone to a small series of men with advanced obstructing prostate cancer.[3] They found that in acute obstruction, steroids could obviate the need for urinary diversion and its associated complications including infection, bleeding, and dislodgement. Similar results have been seen for metastatic colon cancer.[4] The recommended steroid regimen is an initial dose of 8 mg dexamethasone intravenously, followed by different doses and frequencies as listed in Table 11.1. Fluids are also restricted until a diuresis becomes apparent. The results are usually rapid and may be evident within 72 h. Nearly 90% of patients in these studies experienced dramatic improvement in their acute renal failure and were able to avoid urinary diversion. However, nearly half of these failed to respond to definitive treatment and died 3–4 weeks after the high dose steroids were stopped.

Intervention

Once the diagnosis, level of obstruction and cause have been established, varying degrees of intervention may be appropriate. Drainage procedures can be palliative or definitive. The level of obstruction usually dictates the best method of intervention. In bladder outlet obstruction, placement of a urinary

Table 11.1 Dexamethasone regimen

Day	Dose (mg)	Frequency (hourly)	Method
0	8	–	IV
1–3	4	6	IV
3–6	4	8	oral
6–9	4	12	oral
9–12	2	8	oral
12–22	2	12	oral
22–28	2	24	oral

catheter may be sufficient, and where this in not possible, suprapubic catheterization may be performed. These drainage techniques may be used as an emergency to relieve obstruction until surgery or chemotherapy can be performed to reduce tumour mass, but can also be used as long-term solutions. Use of haemofiltration or dialysis may be necessary and can be performed using triple lumen necklines in the short term.

Nephrostomy Percutaneous nephrostomy insertion is one option for supra-vesical obstruction. The technique can be used for unilateral and bilateral ureteric obstruction. Initial puncture of the collecting system can be performed under ultrasound guidance and using local anaesthesia. As it avoids the need for general anaesthesia, this technique may be of particular help in the management of patients with abnormal biochemistry or in a poor physical state, in particular those patients with hyperkalaemia or heart failure.

After the initial puncture of the collecting system, contrast material can be injected to image the collecting system and a nephrostomy tube is inserted using a modified 'Seldinger' technique. Urine collected from the collecting system should be cultured and the procedure covered with antibiotics active against common urinary tract pathogens (mainly Gram-negative bacilli).

After decompression of the collecting system, the nephrostomy can be used for injection of contrast to image the level and nature of the obstruction. Antegrade passage of a guide wire across the obstruction may be used to place an indwelling stent. This technique has the advantage that the nephrostomy tube can subsequently be removed, thus improving the patients comfort. If antegrade stent placement is not possible, long-term nephrostomy drainage is feasible over many months and in some cases, years. The nephrostomy tube may become blocked by sediment in long-term usage. Passage of a guidewire down the lumen of the stent (under X-ray screening) or change of the nephrostomy over a guidewire may be necessary.

The main complications of nephrostomy drainage are haemorrhage, infection, and displacement of the tube. A variety of locking devices to maintain the intra-renal loop of tubing and external fixation techniques have reduced the incidence of accidental displacement following successful insertion.

Stents

The use of self-retaining ureteric stents (often called 'J' or 'double J' stents) is a useful alternative to nephrostomy drainage for supra-vesical obstruction. The main advantage is that they are 'internal' and do not necessitate any external tubing. The normal (retrograde) method of placement is via the bladder using a cystoscope to introduce a guidewire into the ureter, passed the obstruction and into the renal pelvis. The stent is then passed over the guidewire and its position checked using an image intensifier. In some patients in whom the ureteric obstruction is either very narrow or tortuous, it may not be possible to pass a conventional guidewire. The development of hydrophilic guidewires, which become extremely slippery when in contact with fluid, have revolutionised the ability to introduce stents for such challenging patients. Difficult ureteric strictures may need to be managed with a combined retrograde and antegrade approach where a guidewire can be passed from above, grasped from below and a stent inserted after dilatation of the obstruction. Under normal circumstances, a rigid cystoscope is used with the patient under general or regional anaesthesia. Stents can be inserted using flexible cystoscopes under local anaesthesia. Stents can also be passed in an antegrade fashion via a nephrostomy tract as described above.

Stents can cause symptoms—usually in the form of irritative urinary symptoms and haematuria. In some patients they induce symptoms similar to ureteric colic and become intolerable. After a variable time in contact with urine, deposits of calcium and phosphate may 'encrust' the surface and obstruct the lumen. Extensive encrustation may interfere with removal of the stent. Encrustation varies in its extent and the speed with which it occurs between different patients. Patients who have a history of urinary stone formation should be monitored carefully with radiography.

Stents are usually, but not always, successful in relieving ureteric obstruction, especially when renal function is preserved in the affected kidney. Obstruction of the ureter over a long distance and very poor renal function may militate against a sufficient 'pressure drop' to enable the stent to function. Experimental studies have revealed that urine may pass around the stent to a greater extent than traverse the lumen. If the patient fails to improve after stent placement, they should be re-assessed and an alternative drainage method considered.

The choice of nephrostomy or stent is much debated and depends on the patient's condition and the obstructing lesion. The choice of drainage method may also be dictated by the skills of the available personnel.

Surgical urinary diversion

Placement of stents and insertion of nephrostomy tubes can be seen as temporary methods of overcoming obstructive uropathy. In the acute presentation, they allow for immediate relief of obstruction and treatment of associated infection. Once the patient's condition has been stabilized, then it is necessary to consider longer term management. For those patients who have a limited prognosis and others who are not able, or willing, to undergo further 'definitive procedures', they can be used for longer-term management. A schedule should be drawn up to show when changes of the stent or nephrostomy are required.

Where possible, the temporary relief should be followed by definitive relief of the obstruction. The precise procedure will depend on the nature and site of the obstruction. Obstruction in the distal ureter can be overcome by re-implantation of the ureter, which may involve creation of a tubularized bladder flap (such as the Boari flap) to bridge a defect. In the mid-ureter, it may be possible to excise the obstruction and mobilse the ureter to allow an end-to-end anastomosis. An alternative is to use healthy ureter from the affected side and swing it across to anastomose to the other ureter—the trans-uretero-ureterostomy. Interposition of appendix or small bowel may be necessary to bridge long defects in the ureter.

Bilateral lower ureteric obstruction may be best managed by complete diversion of the urinary stream from the bladder. The healthy proximal ureters can be joined together and anastomosed to an isolated segment of small bowel to form an ileal conduit, which is brought to the surface as a urostomy.

When circumstances are dire, and this is usually associated with other problems such as fistula or sepsis, one method of management of unilateral obstruction, is to perform a nephrectomy or to deprive the affected kidney of its blood supply using trans-catheter arterial embolization.

Post-obstructive diuresis

Relief of obstruction will usually result in a large diuresis and a temporary salt-losing nephropathy may ensue. A massive polyuria causing litres of urine to be produced may be seen particularly after catheterization for bladder outlet obstruction. It is usually less marked following relief of unilateral renal obstruction. Major salts lost are K, Na, and Cl, and other ions (Mg, Ca, PO_4, and HCO_3 may be lost to a lesser degree). Intravenous fluid replacement is essential for major loses but should be cautiously reduced after 24 h, as it may perpetuate diuresis. Most authors advocate 0.45% saline for fluid replacement, although 0.9% saline may also be used and is usually more readily available. Fluid replacement should aim to replace all urinary loses for the first 24 h and once renal function has been seen to improve may be weaned appropriately thereafter. Frequent monitoring of vital signs, weight and urine output are critical and renal function biochemistry may need to be checked more than once a day. In cases of major urinary loses with derangement of biochemical values, it may be necessary to add K, Mg, Ca, or HCO_3 to intravenous fluids.

Prognosis

The rate at which irreversible kidney damage occurs in urinary tract obstruction is dependant upon four factors:

1. The degree of obstruction.
2. The duration of obstruction. Complete obstruction for a period of weeks will result in only partial return to normal renal function. Complete obstruction for months usually results in irreversible damage. A better outcome is seen in partial obstruction depending upon the degree of obstruction and duration.
3. The level of obstruction. Obstruction occurring at the bladder neck may often induce detrusor hypertrophy protecting the kidneys by avoiding a rise in pressure in the upper urinary tracts.
4. Supervening infection. Ascending infections of the urinary tract usually induced by stasis or instrumentation and rapidly induces irreversible renal necrosis.

Relieving ureteric obstruction in a woman with advanced malignancy can transform her outlook as difficult symptoms are brought under control. The prognosis of the underlying disease will usually determine the outcome for the patient in the longer term: if the woman has very advanced disease and is generally deteriorating, interventional treatment may not be appropriate. It is essential that the patient's goals guide the direction of treatment but she needs to be informed of all the possible options available to her. Care of the patient with advanced pelvic malignancy involves teamwork, with other specialists in primary and secondary care, whose contributions are covered in other chapters in this book.

References

1 Bosch, A., Frias, Z., and Valda, G. C. (1973). Prognostic significance of ureteral obstruction in carcinoma of cervix uteri. *Acta Radiol Ther Phys Biol*, **12**(1), 47–56.
2 Lau, K. O., Hia, T. N., Cheng, C., and Tay, S. K. (1998). Outcome of obstructive uropathy after pelvic irradiation in patients with carcinoma of uterine cervix. *Ann Acad Med Singapore*, **27**(5), 631–5.
3 Hamdy, F. C. and Williams, J. L. (1995). Use of dexamethasone for ureteric obstruction in advanced prostate cancer: use of percutaneous nephrostomies can be avoided. *Br J Urol*, **75**(6), 782–5.
4 Chye, R. and Lickiss, N. (1994). The use of corticosteroids in the management of bilateral malignant ureteric obstruction. *J Pain & Sympt Manage*, **9**(8), 537–40.

Chapter 12

The last days of life

John Ellershaw

For women who develop incurable gynaecological cancer, the journey they experience can be complex. They may undergo both curative and palliative treatments, which can include surgery, radiotherapy, and chemotherapy. They often live with uncertainty. Sometimes they may feel well and at other times they may feel very ill. Psychologically they may have to deal with the implications of a foreshortened life. They will lose relationships that they expected would continue for many years. If they have young children, they will feel this loss even more acutely.

Despite our best efforts to palliate both the disease and its symptoms, patients with incurable cancer will sooner or later enter the dying phase; that is, the last hours/days of life. This phase of care will be the focus of this chapter. It will examine developments in care, not only for the patient, but for those who are close to them.

Diagnosing dying

Whether the patient is in hospital or in the community, it is important that the healthcare team caring for them recognize the dying phase, i.e. that they are able to 'diagnose dying'. This is an essential skill, which will ensure good symptom control, and appropriate psychosocial and spiritual support for the patient and their family. However, there are a number of factors that may act as barriers to healthcare teams diagnosing dying:

◆ In some circumstances, active treatment is continued when there is little or no clinical response. It is not recognized that the treatment has become futile and is causing more harm than benefit to the patient.

◆ In situations where there is no definitive diagnosis, or a new symptom has arisen without an obvious cause, the decision to undertake investigations may create a wait of several days before results are available. This continued pursuit of clinical causation can draw attention away from the patient's overall deterioration.

◆ The patient and their family may be aware that the situation is continuing to deteriorate. If they feel that this is not being recognized and discussed with them, their trust in the healthcare professionals may be eroded.

◆ There are key skills, knowledge, and attitudes, which are essential in the care of the dying, and if the team are not trained in these areas they will not feel competent at dealing with symptom control, communicating appropriately, and meeting the needs of the patient and family in the dying phase. This may result in a distressing death for the patient, and leave the family unsupported and possibly angry and resentful at the level of care received.

◆ Ethical issues, such as resuscitation status and discontinuing inappropriate medication and hydration, can also influence care at the end of life in a detrimental way if not addressed.

◆ The cultural and spiritual needs of dying patients are diverse. However, living in a pluralistic society often normalizes some of this. At certain points in life, including at the time of death, this diversity is often accentuated, so that religious practices and customs become important to the patient and their family. These must be understood and facilitated by the healthcare team. Fear or ignorance of these issues can prevent a diagnosis of dying from being made, resulting in a distressing, unplanned death for the patient.

◆ Some women dying of gynaecological malignancy may have unresolved issues about their fertility—particularly if they have not borne children and have had their uterus removed in the course of the treatment, which, it was hoped, would cure them.

If a patient dies an undignified death in pain or agitation, or if the relatives have been unsupported and poorly informed regarding the condition of their loved one, there are a number of potential consequences. First, the relatives may be shocked by what has happened and then become angry at the care of their loved one. Such distressing memories can lead to complex bereavement issues. Second, the healthcare professionals involved with the patient can feel as if they have failed the patient and delivered poor medical and nursing care. It is therefore important that we diagnose the dying phase and have a structure in place for the care of dying patients and their families. This structure will now be explored in more depth.

The signs and symptoms of dying—diagnosing dying

There are occasions when the dying phase for a cancer patient can be precipitous; for example, they may have a massive haemorrhage. However, it is more usually preceded by a gradual deterioration in functional status, accompanied by a decreased intake of food and fluid. In cancer patients the following signs are commonly associated with the dying phase:

- the patient becomes bed-bound;
- the patient is semi-comatose;
- the patient is only able to take sips of fluid;
- the patient is no longer able to take oral medication.[1]

A major shift in thinking for the clinical team is needed in order to move away from investigation and treatment regarding the disease process, and towards a focus on symptom control for the patient. Once the dying phase has been identified it is important to consider where the patient herself would prefer to be during this time. She may have indicated that she would prefer to die at home, in a hospice, or in hospital. There must be a reassessment of the patient's needs, which includes the physical, psychological, social, and spiritual aspects of care.

Place of death

Over the last century there has been an increasing shift towards patients dying in hospital rather than at home. For example, in the UK over 50% of all cancer deaths occur in hospital.[2] This is due in part to the complex nature of the disease and the investigations and treatments that patients undergo in the last months of life. It also reflects the challenges of providing adequate social and practical support at home for the dying patient. If a patient expresses the wish to die at home, then procedures should be in place to enable the patient either to remain at home or to be transferred home if she is in hospital. For this to be achieved, good communication between the hospital and community teams is essential, as is 24-h access to drugs in the community and ideally access to a 24-h nursing service. For some patients dying at home neither is possible, practical, nor wished for by the patient. For patients who do not wish to die at home or in a hospital there is an alternative. Since the 1950s hospices have been developing specialist expertise in care of the dying, and for 15% of patients in the UK with cancer, the hospice has provided an alternative place of death to home or hospital.[3–5]

Anticipatory planning

With modern medical and nursing expertise, it should be possible for patients to die a peaceful and dignified death and their relatives should be adequately supported. In order to achieve these outcomes of care, anticipatory planning is important. Once the patient is diagnosed as dying and the place of care identified, the needs of the patient and family over the next hours and days can be

Table 12.1 Goals of care for patients in the dying phase (Adapted from the Liverpool Care Pathway for the Dying Patient—Initial Assessment)

COMFORT MEASURES

GOAL 1: Current medication assessed and non essentials discontinued

GOAL 2: As required subcutaneous medication written up as per protocol (pain, agitation, respiratory tract secretions, nausea, and vomiting)

GOAL 3: Discontinue inappropriate interventions (blood tests, antibiotics, intravenous fluids/medications—not for cardiopulmonary resuscitation documented, turning regimes/vital signs)

....

PSYCHOLOGICAL/INSIGHT

GOAL 4: Ability to communicate in English assessed as adequate (translator not needed)

GOAL 5: Insight into condition assessed

....

RELIGIOUS/SPIRITUAL SUPPORT

GOAL 6: Religious/spiritual needs assessed with patient/family

....

COMMUNICATION WITH FAMILY/OTHER

GOAL 7: Identify how family/other are to be informed of patients impending death

GOAL 8: Family/other given relevant hospital information

....

COMMUNICATION WITH PRIMARY HEALTH CARE TEAM

GOAL 9: General practitioner is aware of patient's condition

....

SUMMARY

GOAL 10: Plan of care explained and discussed with patient/family

GOAL 11: Family/other express understanding of plan of care

---

anticipated (Table 12.1).[6] In order for these needs to be met, it is important that the healthcare team is proactive in their approach. This proactive model of care is contrary to the withdrawal that sometimes occurs in the hospital setting.[7] Healthcare professionals require specific training in this area to enable them to provide the highest standards of care for the patient. The goals of care associated with care of the dying will now be discussed in more detail.

Physical care

As the patient's condition deteriorates and they become weaker, it becomes increasingly difficult for them to take oral medication. Therefore it is important to discontinue non-essential medication, e.g. anti-hypertensives or diuretics, and continue via a parenteral route those drugs that are essential for symptom control. These include analgesics, anxiolytics, drugs for control of respiratory tract secretions, and anti-emetics.

Conversion of oral morphine to subcutaneous diamorphine or morphine is shown in Table 12.2. If the patient has an epidural or intrathecal delivery mechanism for pain control this should generally be continued in the dying phase. The patient should also be prescribed as required (PRN) subcutaneous medication for pain, agitation, and respiratory tract secretions (Table 12.3). Medication during the dying phase is often administered by the subcutaneous route. If the patient needs regular medication this is best delivered by a continuous subcutaneous infusion via a syringe driver.

A combination of drugs can be mixed in the syringe and this is slowly infused usually over a 24-h period. It is important to check compatibilities before mixing drugs.[8]

The issue of discontinuing futile investigations and treatments has already been discussed. This also embraces what may be perceived as routine interventions in a hospital setting, e.g. blood tests, routine turning regimens, and measuring vital signs. Discontinuing some interventions may need greater discussion within the team. For example, sometimes continuation of antibiotics can be justified if it will improve symptom control. Otherwise they should be discontinued in the dying phase. Evidence is limited but suggests that the continuation of artificial hydration in dying patients is of limited benefit and, in general, artificial hydration can be discontinued in the dying phase. If it is to be continued, the maximum recommended is 1 litre of fluid over 24 h. The symptoms that can be related to hydration in this phase of care, particularly dry mouth, are often best relieved by local measures and family members can be encouraged to participate in this type of care.[9]

The issue of cardiopulmonary resuscitation is increasingly discussed with patients and their families. It is an area that needs to be dealt with in a sensitive manner, but in the same way as burdensome treatments and interventions are withdrawn at this phase of life, the futile intervention of cardiopulmonary resuscitation should not be undertaken in the dying patient.[10]

Following the initial re-focusing of care, the patient needs continuing assessment of their physical care. The patient may complain of pain directly, or may grimace or have localized tenderness when moved, indicating the need for additional analgesia. In the dying phase, the patient's renal function may deteriorate and opioid accumulation may occur. This may be clinically observed as myoclonic jerks. This is an infrequent occurrence and is generally not distressing to the patient. However, if the myoclonic jerks are frequent and troublesome, a dose reduction in the opioid is indicated. At times, distinguishing between pain and agitation can be difficult but in patients who are restless and agitated, appropriate anxiolytics should be administered. The treatment of respiratory tract secretions with antimuscarinic agents is common within palliative care.

Table 12.2 Prescribing diamorphine and morphine for care of the dying

	As required (PRN) medication	Opioids for administration by continuous subcutaneous infusion over 24 h
Diamorphine	1. Patient not on regular opioid: Diamorphine 2.5–5 mg subcutaneous 4-hourly 2. Patient on opioid subcutaneous infusion: Dose of Diamorphine should be 1/6 of 24-h dose in syringe driver e.g. diamorphine 30 mg subcutaneous via driver will require 5 mg diamorphine subcutaneous 4 hourly	To convert a patient from oral Diamorphine to a 24-h subcutaneous infusion of diamorphine divide the total daily dose of diamorphine by three e.g. MST 30 mg b.d. orally = diamorphine 20 mg via subcutaneous infusion over 24 h
Morphine	1. Patient not on regular opioid: Morphine 2.5–5 mg subcutaneous 4-hourly 2. Patient on opioid subcutaneous infusion: Dose of morphine should be 1/6 of 24-h dose in syringe driver e.g. morphine 30 mg subcutaneous via driver will require 5 mg morphine subcutaneous 4-hourly	To convert a patient from oral morphine to a 24-h subcutaneous infusion of diamorphine divide the total daily dose of morphine by two e.g. MST 30 mg b.d. orally = morphine 30 mg via subcutaneous infusion over 24 h

Table 12.3 Drugs commonly used for symptom control in care of the dying

	As required (PRN) medication	Usual total daily dose—including CSCI and PRN medication
Anti-emetic	Cyclizine 50 mg 8-hourly Metoclopramide 10 mg 6-hourly Levomepromazine 6.25 mg 8-hourly Haloperidol 1.5 mg 8-hourly	Cyclizine 75–150 mg daily Metoclopramide 30–120 mg daily Levomepromazine 6.25–25 mg daily Haloperidol 5–10 mg daily
Sedative	*Midazolam 2.5–5 mg 4-hourly *Levomepromazine 6.25–12.5 mg 8-hourly	Midazolam 10–60 mg daily Levomepromazine 25–200 mg daily
Control of respiratory tract secretions	Glycopyrronium 0.2 mg 4-hourly Hyoscine butylbromide 20 mg 4-hourly Hyoscine hydrobromide 0.4 mg 4-hourly	Glycopyrronium 0.6–1.2 mg Hyoscine butylbromide 20–60 mg Hyoscine hydrobromide 1.2–2.4 mg

* As required PRN dose may need increasing if patient on regular subcutaneous infusion over 24 h.

Although there is only limited research evidence in this area, what there is suggests that early treatment leads to more effective management of this symptom.

It is also important that the patient's mouth is kept moist and clean with at least four-hourly mouth care, although this can be given more frequently if necessary. Relatives can be involved in this area enabling them to make a direct contribution to the care of their loved one.

Incontinence may cause problems in ongoing care for the dying patient. This can be relieved by catheterization. Urinary retention may also occur in this phase and any patient who becomes acutely agitated should be clinically examined to exclude a distended bladder. Again this is an indication for catheterization of patients in the dying phase. Bowel intervention is rarely necessary in the last days and hours of life. There may be other specific needs regarding physical care; for example, fungating wounds and pressure areas, which will require continued attention in this phase. It is important that any intervention undertaken is primarily aimed at the comfort of the patient and does not cause unnecessary distress.

In order to maintain good symptom control in the dying phase it is important that patients have ready access to 'as required' medication for pain, agitation, and respiratory tract secretions.

Anticipatory prescribing by the ward ensures this ease of access. In the community, trained nurses are needed to facilitate access to 'as required' medication for families and carers of patients.

Psychological care

The importance of good communication skills to manage this phase of life well, has been mentioned a number of times.[11] These skills include:

♦ Being able to break bad news; the family need to understand clearly that the patient is now in the dying phase.

♦ Dealing with difficult questions, e.g. the patient may want to know why no further treatment is being undertaken.

♦ Addressing existential questions, such as 'why me?', 'why now?'.

♦ Giving information in a clear and sensitive manner regarding previous interventions and outcomes of treatment.

It is also very important that the needs of children should be addressed when a parent or close relative is dying. There is a danger that children can be marginalized at this sensitive time and so it is important to recognize their needs and their level of awareness regarding issues of death and dying (see Table 12.4).

Table 12.4 Stages of children's grief

Age range	Concept of death	Possible behaviours
Up to 3 years	No understanding of death	Regression Feeding and sleeping patterns disrupted Anxiety due to separation from carer/parent
3–5 years	Death seen as reversible—person will return May feel they have caused the death by misbehaving 'Magical' thinking—therefore easy to believe that death is temporary	Sadness, anxiety, fear of losing other parent/carer Persistent crying, screaming Reluctance to accept changes in day to day activities Problems sleeping Regression
5–11 years	More cognitive understanding of death	Withdrawal, sadness, loneliness, depression Anger Fear of own mortality Perfect child Regression Brave—masking emotions Difficulties at school
Teenagers	Understanding of finality of death Denial—not wanting to believe that it has happened	Withdrawal, sadness, depression, loneliness Adopting responsibilities of deceased parent Anger rejection Fear of own mortality Joking sarcasm Regression Guilt—relationship with parent before death

It is important when assessing the insight of the patient and family that this is done on a regular basis, as information may need repeating or further explanation may be necessary because it has been misinterpreted or not clearly understood. There may also be a number of family members all of whom may need to hear the same information. As the dying phase progresses and the patient becomes comatose, the main focus for good communication becomes the relatives. It is important to use unambiguous language, and to reinforce to the relative that the patient is now dying, so that they clearly understand the situation. Sometimes relatives who have previously wanted only a little information and may have been in some form of 'denial', now need to be confronted with the reality of the situation. It is a constant source of frustration and anger voiced by bereaved relatives that no-one sat down with them and discussed the fact that their loved one was dying. This discussion gives the family an opportunity to ask any questions they may have. It allows them time to decide the best way to manage the last days and hours of life, and to consider how to say goodbye to their loved one. It also gives them time to contact and inform other people who may be important to the patient. Clear, consistent, and sensitive communication is essential to prepare the family for the death of the patient.

Social care

In order that the patient receives optimum care and the family receives good support in the dying phase, social and practical care is essential. This will depend on the setting. In hospital it is important to ensure that the family are made aware of the facilities available to support them; for example, whether they can stay overnight and where they can get food and drink. They need to know how they can gain access to the hospital if they are called back in the middle of the night urgently. An information sheet, which can be given to relatives at this time, is an effective way to reinforce verbal communication.

In the community, the family may need increased practical support in the home. This can range from 24-h nursing care to a contact telephone number where they can get help and advice on a 24-h basis. They also need information on what to do if the patient dies and a healthcare professional is not present. This information and practical support is essential if families are to be given a feeling of control at this very emotional and demanding time.

Spiritual care

Sensitivity to the patient's cultural and religious background is essential. This may require formal religious traditions to be observed in the dying phase, and may influence care of the body after death.[12] In the hospital setting, access to information and support from the various religious and spiritual traditions is essential to meet the needs of patients in the dying phase. This information needs to be co-ordinated and made available at ward level. In the patient's home it is often a local contact familiar to the family who will support them at this time.

Bereavement care

Following the patient's death, relatives should be dealt with in a compassionate manner. They are often at their most vulnerable at this time and need clear concise information regarding the practical procedures that must be followed. A bereavement leaflet explaining issues relating to grief can also be helpful. The key areas that this should embrace are:

- The mixed emotions that may be felt including that of shock, disbelief, and guilt, which may be associated with anger about what has happened or what did not happen with the patient's care, or the bereaved's relationship with the deceased.

- The issue of depression should be included and the fact that it is important to link with the primary healthcare team should this feeling persist.

The needs of bereaved children should also be addressed. Children under the age of four are generally best supported by their parents or carer, due to the issue of separation anxiety. Above that age children are still best supported by their parent or carer. If, however, there are physical or emotional reasons why this is not possible, some level of therapeutic intervention may be appropriate.[13, 14]

It is important to bear in mind that for some, grief may take months to come to terms with, while for others it may take years. However, with time and the appropriate support, the memories will become less painful and life will start to rebuild itself.[15]

It is essential to inform the GP/family physician when the patient dies, and give any important information about the manner of her death. The family will be supported and cared for in the community when they leave the hospital. If the relatives are not registered with the patient's GP and you have concerns about them, you will need to obtain their permission to pass these onto their own doctor.

Providing a framework of care

It is a key aim of specialist palliative care to disseminate best practice for dying patients among all healthcare professionals. An expanding educational programme at undergraduate and postgraduate level aims to empower generic healthcare workers. Integrated care pathways are one way to provide a framework of care.[6, 16] This can incorporate guidance for practice regarding:

- making the diagnosis of dying;
- initial assessment and care;
- ongoing care;
- care after death.

This type of model can integrate evidence-based practice and guidelines into practice. It can also encourage team-working and facilitate a peaceful dignified death for the patient with support for the relatives.

Conclusion

For women with gynaecological cancer, the dying phase is important. The last days and hours of the patient's life will become some of the lasting memories for the families and, in particular, their children. It is therefore incumbent on the healthcare professionals caring for women with widespread progressive disease to diagnose dying, so that the best possible care can be facilitated at the earliest possible stage. This includes identifying the preferred place to die, ensuring that anticipatory care regarding physical, psychological, social, and spiritual needs are met, and that, following the patient's death, appropriate bereavement care is available for the family. Using frameworks of care to empower the generic team is an important step forward in this area of care, together with the appropriate use of specialist palliative care services. However, perhaps the most important lesson for healthcare professionals, who are striving to provide the best possible care for the dying, comes from a husband whose wife died in distress who said, 'all the excellent treatment she had before meant nothing because she died a painful, undignified death'.

References

1 Ellershaw, J. E., Sutcliffe, J., and Saunders, C. M. (1995). The dying patient and dehydration. *Journal of Pain and Symptom Management*, **10**(3), 192–197.

2 ONS Office of National Statistics (2000). *http://www.statistics.gov.uk*

3 Twycross, R. and Lichter, I. (1998). The terminal phase. In *Oxford book of palliative medicine*, 2nd edn (Doyle, D., Hanks, G. W. C., and MacDonald, N., ed.), pp. 995–997. Oxford University Press, Oxford.

4 Working Party on Clinical Guidelines in Palliative Care (1997). *Changing gear: guidelines for managing the last days of life: the research evidence*. National Council for Hospice and Specialist Palliative Care Services.

5 Ellershaw, J. E., Smith, C., Overill, S., Walker, S. E., and Aldridge, J. (2001). Care of the dying: Setting standards for symptom control in the last 48 hours of life. *Journal of Pain and Symptom Management*, **21**(1), 12–17.

6 Ellershaw, J. E., Murphy, D., Shea, T., Foster, A., and Overill, S. (1997). Development of a multiprofessional care pathway for the dying patient. *European Journal of Palliative Care*, **4**(6), 203–208.

7 Glare, P. (1998). Palliative care in teaching hospitals:achievement or aberration? *Progress in Palliative Care*, **6**(1), 4–9.

8 Dickman, A., Littlewood, C., and Varga, J. (2002). *The syringe driver*. Oxford University Press, Oxford.

9 Joint Working Party between the National Council for Hospice and Specialist Palliative Care Services and the Ethics Committee of the Association for Palliative Medicine of Great Britain and Ireland (1997). Ethical decision making in palliative care: artificial hydration for people who are terminally ill. *Journal of the European Association of Palliative Care*, July/August, 124.

10 Joint Working Party between the National Council for Hospice and Specialist Palliative Care Services and the Ethics Committee of the Association for Palliative Medicine of Great Britain and Ireland (2002). *Ethical decision making in palliative care: cardiopulmonary resuscitation for people who are terminally ill*. National Council for Hospice and Specialist Palliative Care Services.

11 Fallowfield, L. J., Jenkins, V. A., and Beveridge, H. A. (2002). Truth may hurt but deceit hurts more: communication in palliative care. *Palliative Medicine*, **16**, 297–303.

12 Neuberger, J. (1999). *Caring for dying people of different faiths*. Butterworth-Heinemann.

13 Worden, W. (1996). *Children and grief*. Guildford Press, Guildford.

14 Silverman, P. (1999). *Never too young to know*. Oxford University Press, Oxford.

15 Worden, J. W. (1982). *Grief counselling and grief therapy*. Tavistock/Routledge, London.

16 Bookbinder, M. and Romer, A. L. (2002). Raising the standard of care for imminently dying patients. *Journal of Palliative Medicine*, **5**(4), 635–645.

Index

Printed in the United Kingdom
by Lightning Source UK Ltd.
132633UK00002BA/5/A

9 780198 528067